Office-Based Surgery in Otolaryngology

Editors

MELISSA A. PYNNONEN
CECELIA E. SCHMALBACH

OTOLARYNGOLOGIC CLINICS OF NORTH AMERICA

www.oto.theclinics.com

Consulting Editor
SUJANA S. CHANDRASEKHAR

June 2019 • Volume 52 • Number 3

ELSEVIER

1600 John F. Kennedy Boulevard • Suite 1800 • Philadelphia, Pennsylvania, 19103-2899

http://www.oto.theclinics.com

OTOLARYNGOLOGIC CLINICS OF NORTH AMERICA Volume 52, Number 3
June 2019 ISSN 0030-6665, ISBN-13: 978-0-323-67846-9

Editor: Jessica McCool
Developmental Editor: Laura Kavanaugh

Otolaryngologic Clinics of North America (ISSN 0030-6665) is published bimonthly by Elsevier, Inc., 360 Park Avenue South, New York, NY 10010-1710. Months of issue are February, April, June, August, October, and December. Business and Editorial Offices: 1600 John F. Kennedy Blvd., Suite 1800, Philadelphia, PA 19103-2899. Customer Service Office: 6277 Sea Harbor Drive, Orlando, FL 32887-4800. Periodicals postage paid at New York, NY and additional mailing offices. Subscription prices are $412.00 per year (US individuals), $889.00 per year (US institutions), $100.00 per year (US student/resident), $548.00 per year (Canadian individuals), $1127.00 per year (Canadian institutions), $564.00 per year (international individuals), $1127.00 per year (international institutions), $270.00 per year (international & Canadian student/resident). Foreign air speed delivery is included in all *Clinics'* subscription prices. All prices are subject to change without notice. **POSTMASTER:** Send address changes to *Otolaryngologic Clinics of North America*, Elsevier Health Sciences Division, Subscription Customer Service, 3251 Riverport Lane, Maryland Heights, MO 63043. **Telephone: 1-800-654-2452 (U.S. and Canada); 314-447-8871 (outside U.S. and Canada). Fax: 314-447-8029. E-mail: journalscustomerservice-usa@elsevier.com (for print support); journalsonlinesupport-usa@elsevier.com (for online support).**

Reprints. For copies of 100 or more of articles in this publication, please contact the Commercial Reprints Department, Elsevier Inc., 360 Park Avenue South, New York, NY 10010-1710. Tel.: 212-633-3874; Fax: 212-633-3820; E-mail: reprints@elsevier.com.

Otolaryngologic Clinics of North America is also published in Spanish by McGraw-Hill Interamericana Editores S.A., P.O. Box 5-237, 06500 Mexico D.F., Mexico.

Otolaryngologic Clinics of North America is covered in *MEDLINE/PubMed (Index Medicus), Current Contents/Clinical Medicine, Excerpta Medica, BIOSIS, Science Citation Index,* and *ISI/BIOMED.*

Contributors

CONSULTING EDITOR

SUJANA S. CHANDRASEKHAR, MD
Past President, American Academy of Otolaryngology–Head and Neck Surgery, Partner, ENT & Allergy Associates, LLP, Clinical Professor, Department of Otolaryngology–Head and Neck Surgery, Zucker School of Medicine at Hofstra-Northwell, Hempstead, New York; Clinical Associate Professor, Department of Otolaryngology–Head and Neck Surgery, Icahn School of Medicine at Mount Sinai, New York, New York

EDITORS

MELISSA A. PYNNONEN, MD, MSc
Professor of Otolaryngology, University of Michigan Health System, Medical Director, West Ann Arbor Health Center, Ann Arbor, Michigan

CECELIA E. SCHMALBACH, MD, MSc, FACS
David Myers, MD Professor and Chair of Otolaryngology–Head and Neck Surgery, Lewis Katz School of Medicine at Temple University, Philadelphia, Pennsylvania

AUTHORS

ABDULMALIK S. ALSAIED, MD
Department of Otolaryngology, Voice, Airway and Swallowing Center, Medical College of Georgia at Augusta University, Augusta, Georgia

DOUGLAS CHIEFFE, MD
Resident, Department of Otolaryngology, University of Minnesota, Minneapolis, Minnesota

MARTIN J. CITARDI, MD
Professor and Chairman, Department of Otorhinolaryngology–Head and Neck Surgery, McGovern Medical School, The University of Texas Health Science Center at Houston, Houston, Texas

MARC DEAN, MD
Chairman, Vitruvio Institute for Medical Advancement, Assistant Clinical Professor, Texas Tech University Health Science Center, Lubbock, Texas

LARA DEVGAN, MD, MPH, FACS
Board-Certified Plastic and Reconstructive Surgeon, Diplomate, American Board of Plastic Surgery, PLLC Plastic & Reconstructive Surgery, New York, New York

GREGORY R. DION, MD, MS
Assistant Professor, Dental and Craniofacial Trauma Research Department, US Army Institute of Surgical Research, JBSA Fort Sam Houston, San Antonio, Texas

KAMALA DURAIRAJ
Georgetown University, Washington, DC

MANUELA FINA, MD
Assistant Professor, Department of Otolaryngology, University of Minnesota,
Minneapolis, Minnesota

ANDREW W. JOSEPH, MD, MPH
Assistant Professor, Facial Plastic and Reconstructive Surgery, Department of
Otolaryngology–Head and Neck Surgery, University of Michigan Medical School,
Ann Arbor, Michigan

SHANNON S. JOSEPH, MD
Assistant Professor, Department of Ophthalmology and Visual Sciences, University of
Michigan Medical School, Ann Arbor, Michigan

DIPTI KAMANI, MD
Division of Thyroid and Parathyroid Surgery, Department of Otolaryngology,
Massachusetts Eye and Ear, Harvard Medical School, Boston, Massachusetts

RICHARD KAO, MD
Department of Otolaryngology–Head and Neck Surgery, Indiana University School of
Medicine, Indianapolis, Indiana

AMBER U. LUONG, MD, PhD
Associate Professor, Department of Otorhinolaryngology–Head and Neck Surgery,
McGovern Medical School, The University of Texas Health Science Center at Houston,
Houston, Texas

SKYLER W. NIELSEN, DO
Department of Otolaryngology–Head and Neck Surgery, Brooke Army Medical Center,
JBSA Fort Sam Houston, San Antonio, Texas

GREGORY N. POSTMA, MD
Department of Otolaryngology, Voice, Airway and Swallowing Center, Medical College of
Georgia at Augusta University, Augusta, Georgia

MELISSA A. PYNNONEN, MD, MSc
Professor of Otolaryngology, University of Michigan Health System, Medical Director,
West Ann Arbor Health Center, Ann Arbor, Michigan

CYRUS C. RABBANI, MD
Department of Otolaryngology–Head and Neck Surgery, Indiana University School of
Medicine, Indianapolis, Indiana

GREGORY W. RANDOLPH, MD, FACS, FACE
Division of Thyroid and Parathyroid Surgery, Department of Otolaryngology,
Massachusetts Eye and Ear, Division of Surgical Oncology, Endocrine Surgery Service,
Department of Surgery, Massachusetts General Hospital, Harvard Medical School,
Boston, Massachusetts

ALOK T. SAINI, MD
Assistant Professor, Department of Otorhinolaryngology–Head and Neck Surgery,
University of Kentucky College of Medicine, Lexington, Kentucky

CECELIA E. SCHMALBACH, MD, MSc, FACS
David Myers, MD Professor and Chair of Otolaryngology–Head and Neck Surgery, Lewis Katz School of Medicine at Temple University, Philadelphia, Pennsylvania

TAHA Z. SHIPCHANDLER, MD, FACS
Division of Facial Plastic, Aesthetic and Reconstructive Surgery, Department of Otolaryngology–Head and Neck Surgery, Indiana University School of Medicine, Indianapolis, Indiana

LAWRENCE M. SIMON, MD
LSU Health Sciences Center, Clinical Assistant Professor, Department of Otolaryngology–Head and Neck Surgery, University Hospital and Clinics, Lafayette, Louisiana

CHARLES BLAKELY SIMPSON, MD
Director, The University of Texas Voice Center, Brian N. Sheth Distinguished Chair for Voice and Airway Disorders, Professor, Department of Otolaryngology–Head and Neck Surgery, University of Texas Health Science Center at San Antonio, San Antonio, Texas

PRIYANKA SINGH
Princeton University, Princeton, New Jersey

CRISTIAN M. SLOUGH, MD
Willamette Valley Ear, Nose, & Throat, Willamette Valley Medical Center, McMinnville, Oregon

KATHLEEN M. TIBBETTS, MD
Assistant Professor, Department of Otolaryngology–Head and Neck Surgery, University of Texas Southwestern Medical Center, Dallas, Texas

JONATHAN Y. TING, MD
Division of Rhinology, Department of Otolaryngology–Head and Neck Surgery, Indiana University School of Medicine, Indianapolis, Indiana

RICHARD W. WAGUESPACK, MD
Clinical Professor, Department of Otolaryngology–Head and Neck Surgery, The University of Alabama at Birmingham, Birmingham, Alabama

JOHN WHELAN, BSN, RN
Ann Arbor, Michigan

WILLIAM C. YAO, MD
Assistant Professor, Department of Otorhinolaryngology–Head and Neck Surgery, McGovern Medical School, The University of Texas Health Science Center at Houston, Houston, Texas

Contents

Office-based otolaryngology procedures provide a safe and efficient alternative to the traditional operating room. Physicians are responsible for knowing their state regulations and subspecialty guidelines. Although the clinic setting has fewer regulations than hospitals and ambulatory surgery centers, the clinic has the same standards as a hospital with respect to emergency equipment, trained personnel, protocols, and safety measures. Sedation occurs along a continuum; it is impossible to predict a patient's response to sedation. Otolaryngologists performing office-based sedation must be prepared to rescue with airway and advanced life support in the event that the sedation level encountered is deeper than expected.

Reprocessing a flexible endoscope is a complex multistep process. Attention to detail is essential for patient safety. Physicians need to empower their staff to function as guardians and advocates for best practices in endoscope reprocessing. Current best practice standards and guidelines for flexible endoscope reprocessing in the United States have been led by the Society of Gastroenterology Nurses and Associates, the Association for the Advancement of Medical Instrumentation, the Association of peri-Operative Registered Nurses, American Society for Gastrointestinal Endoscopy, and Multisociety Guideline. This article focuses on important aspects and current best practices for flexible endoscope cleaning and high-level disinfection.

This review article provides a summary of current correct coding for in-office surgical procedures. The relevant Current Procedural Terminology codes are covered and tips and guidance provided for their correct use. Also, where applicable, facility versus nonfacility reimbursement policy and the associated implications for physicians practicing in hospital-based clinics are discussed.

OTOLARYNGOLOGIC CLINICS
OF NORTH AMERICA

SERIES OF RELATED INTEREST

Facial Plastic Surgery Clinics
Available at: https://www.facialplastic.theclinics.com/

THE CLINICS ARE AVAILABLE ONLINE!
Access your subscription at:
www.theclinics.com

Foreword

Maximizing Office-based Otolaryngology Care for Better Patient Outcomes

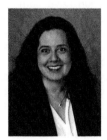

Sujana S. Chandrasekhar, MD, FACS, FAAOHNS
Consulting Editor

It is remarkable to know that, today, a patient can walk in with a complaint, have their otolaryngology problem or cosmetic concern diagnosed, have the corrective treatment performed, and go on to full recovery, without ever having to set foot in an operating room or inpatient setting.

Traditionally, and not so long ago, otolaryngologists provided diagnostic care in the office and took patients to the operating room for any complex diagnostic intervention or surgical procedure. This often involved systemic anesthesia, an overnight stay or longer in the hospital, and significant schedule adjustments and resource allocations. Times have changed. Admission the night before surgery has gone by the wayside. Most routine otolaryngology procedures went to same-day surgery. And now, as knowledge, safety, and instrumentation have improved, a significant number of procedures once reserved for operating rooms are able to be done in the otolaryngologist's office. This saves time, money, anxiety, at times the potential added risks of systemic anesthesia, and reduces possible exposure to pathogens in a hospital.

This issue of *Otolaryngologic Clinics of North America* edited by Drs Pynnonen and Schmalbach is an up-to-date resource for physicians and their office staff on when to offer and how to prepare for and perform office-based surgery for various head and neck disorders. Attention is paid to patient safety concerns and how to minimize risk to the patient and to the care team. As instruments get more complex, maintaining their sterility and reusability does also. The otolaryngologist doing any of the procedures covered in this issue of *Otolaryngologic Clinics of North America* will find clear and comprehensive guidance here.

Every aspect of office-based surgery in otolaryngology is covered. The articles on cosmetic and reconstructive surgery of the face illustrate where minimally invasive,

Otolaryngol Clin N Am 52 (2019) xiii–xiv
https://doi.org/10.1016/j.otc.2019.04.001
0030-6665/19/Published by Elsevier Inc.

nonsurgical methods can be used, where surgical procedures should be offered, and how to streamline the care of the patient for best results. The authors remove any confusion regarding when systemic anesthesia is required. Likewise, the articles on endonasal, sinus, and eustachian tube procedures explain correct patient preparation, dosing, and methods for performing potentially uncomfortable or painful procedures successfully under local anesthesia with good visualization. Endoscopic ear examination and surgery is a relatively new concept, and how much and what can be done in the office is explained clearly. In the patient with a neck mass, using in-office ultrasound saves an extra two visits and the anxiety associated with waiting for results. Laryngeal examination and dysphagia evaluation have come a long way from opposing mirrors and sunlight illumination. Voice and swallow restoration can be accomplished safely in the office, for selected patients. And, of course, ensuring that the work performed is captured, coded, and billed correctly will enable the physician to remain in practice and continue to offer care to others.

As many of the authors point out, performing surgery in an office-based setting requires that the patient, the physician, and the staff be correctly prepared. It is a necessary part of the practicing otolaryngologist's armamentarium to appreciate what can be accomplished in the in-office setting, and to offer the care with which they are comfortable. When this can be accomplished, the benefits to the individual patient and their family, to the physician and their office efficiency, and to reducing the burden of health care costs to society are clear and long-lasting.

Again, I compliment Drs Pynnonen and Schmalbach on helming this comprehensive issue of *Otolaryngologic Clinics of North America* and all the authors on their outstanding work. I learned a great deal from reading this, and I think you will as well.

Sujana S. Chandrasekhar, MD, FACS, FAAOHNS
ENT & Allergy Associates, LLP
18 East 48th Street, 2nd Floor
New York, NY 10017, USA

E-mail address:
ssc@nyotology.com

Preface

Office-based Procedures in Otolaryngology

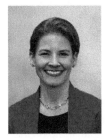
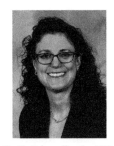

Melissa A. Pynnonen, MD, MSc   Cecelia E. Schmalbach, MD, MSc
Editors

Contemporary otolaryngology clinical practice entails a wide array of office-based surgical procedures. Recent advances in anesthesia, medical technology, and surgical technique have resulted in a shift of procedures from the operating room to the office. Today, 70% of all operations are performed outside the hospital operating room. In fact, it is estimated that up to 15% of procedural interventions occur in an office-based setting.[1]

Office-based surgical procedures provide increased privacy, convenience, and concierge-like service to patients while affording the clinician greater autonomy, flexibility, ease of scheduling, and consistency in working with one's personal staff. Procedures performed in the office are often more efficient and less expensive compared with the operating room. However, the desire for convenience and cost-savings needs to be tempered by the overriding concern for patient safety and consideration of the limited personnel and emergency equipment available in the office.

Office-based procedures range from diagnostic studies involving upper aerodigestive endoscopy and ultrasound-guided needle biopsies to definitive, therapeutic interventions to include laryngeal injections and facial cosmetic procedures. In this issue of *Otolaryngologic Clinics of North America*, we attempt to capture the true breadth and depth of in-office otolaryngology procedures. We include specific articles on laryngology, facial cosmetic surgery, rhinology, otology, head and neck surgery, and reconstruction. Our intention is to stimulate creative thinking among our readers so that we can continuously improve patient-care capabilities. We include an article on coding for office-based procedures, which includes the most current information available. High-level disinfection (HLD), particularly as it pertains to endoscopes, has been heavily scrutinized, and we include a dedicated article on this topic as well as a Standard Operation Procedure (Appendix I) and a medical assistant Competency Assessment (Appendix II) to help the provider facilitate implementation of best practices for HLD

Otolaryngol Clin N Am 52 (2019) xv–xvi
https://doi.org/10.1016/j.otc.2019.03.001
0030-6665/19/© 2019 Published by Elsevier Inc.

in the outpatient clinic. Finally, the same safety standards of a hospital-based operating room must be upheld in the office setting, and we include an article dedicated to patient safety, accreditation, and in-office anesthesia.

We would like to acknowledge the authors, who are truly leading experts in their respective fields. We appreciate the manner in which they shared their experience and associated expertise. We are also indebted to the generation of pioneers who laid the foundation that ultimately led to the office-based otolaryngology procedures used in our daily practice today.

Melissa A. Pynnonen, MD, MSc
University of Michigan Health System
West Ann Arbor Health Center
380 Parkland Plaza
Ann Arbor, MI 48103-6021, USA

Cecelia E. Schmalbach, MD, MSc
Department of Otolaryngology-HNS
Lewis Katz School of Medicine at Temple University
Philadelphia, PA 19140, USA

E-mail addresses:
pynnonen@umich.edu (M.A. Pynnonen)
Cecelia.schmalbach@TUHS.temple.edu (C.E. Schmalbach)

REFERENCE

1. Report of the special committee on outpatient (office-based) surgery. Federation of State Medical Boards. Available at: http://www.fsmb.org/advocacy/policies. Accessed July 1, 2018.

Patient Safety and Anesthesia Considerations for Office-Based Otolaryngology Procedures

Cecelia E. Schmalbach, MD, MSc

KEYWORDS

- Office-based procedures • Local anesthesia • Sedation • Malignant hyperthermia

KEY POINTS

- Otolaryngologists are responsible for remaining current on state regulations and subspecialty society guidelines for office-based procedures.
- The office must maintain the same standards as a hospital with respect to emergency equipment, trained personnel, and safety measures.
- Formal reporting of adverse events and unexpected hospital transfers is highly encouraged by the Federation of State Medical Boards to promote patient safety and quality improvement.
- Sedation is a continuum of 4 levels from anxiolysis alone to general anesthesia.
- Written protocols are warranted for emergencies to include systemic toxicity from local anesthesia, malignant hyperthermia, airway fire, and hospital transfer.

INTRODUCTION

In 1979, fewer than 10% of all surgeries were performed in the outpatient setting. Today, approximately 70% of operations have transferred beyond the confines of a hospital, with 10% to 15% specifically falling into the category of office-based procedures.[1] Advances in anesthesia, surgical technique, and medical technology have allowed for this significant shift. Common office-based otolaryngology procedures are extensive, ranging from cosmetic fillers and facelifts to myringotomy tubes and laryngology procedures.

The first goal of this article is to provide an overview of the accreditation, requirements, and unique considerations to include patient safety, all of which are imperative for successful office-based procedures. The second goal is to provide an overview of anesthetic categories. Local anesthesia options, nerve blocks, and procedural

Disclosure Statement: The author has nothing to disclose.
Otolaryngology–Head and Neck Surgery, Lewis Katz School of Medicine at Temple University, 3440 N, Broad Street, Kresge West, 3rd Floor, Room 309, Philadelphia, PA 19140, USA
E-mail address: Cecelia.Schmalbach@tuhs.temple.edu

Otolaryngol Clin N Am 52 (2019) 379–390
https://doi.org/10.1016/j.otc.2019.02.008
0030-6665/19/© 2019 Elsevier Inc. All rights reserved.

sedation are reviewed with a focus on applications and patient safety. Pertinent information on complications and emergencies are highlighted.

ADVANTAGES AND DISADVANTAGES OF OFFICE-BASED PROCEDURES

Office-based otolaryngology procedures are appealing to both the surgeon and patient for a variety of reasons. Patients often receive increased privacy and greater concierge-like attention in the office compared with larger venues in the hospital or an ambulatory surgery center (ASC). Surgeons have greater autonomy and, therefore, control in their personal office where they can schedule procedures with ease and work with consistent nursing and office staff who are well-versed in their needs, preferences, equipment, and protocols. The office setting provides efficiency and often decreased cost for both the patient and the surgeon.[2]

However, these benefits come with several potential disadvantages related to patient safety. The office setting often provides limited resources to include personnel, equipment, and access to other surgical subspecialists when compared with the traditional hospital operating room or ASC setting. One study using data from the Florida Board of Medicine (2000–2002) specifically compared adverse events and morality between office-based procedures and those conducted at an ASC.[3] The authors reported a 10-fold increase in both patient complications and death for office procedures. They postulate that 43 complications and 6 deaths would have been prevented by conducting the procedures in an ASC.

However, the literature is conflicting. Starling and colleagues[4] published their 10-year prospective study of adverse in-office procedure events in Florida where reporting is mandatory. The authors identified 46 deaths and 263 procedure-related complications warranting hospital transfer. Sixty-seven percent of the deaths and 74% of the complications/hospital transfers were specifically related to elective cosmetic surgery performed under general anesthesia. Similar findings were identified in their 6-year prospective study from Alabama. The authors conclude that office-based procedures are safe and they did not find that accreditation or board certification impacted outcomes. However, the authors continue to champion mandatory reporting. Two additional reviews of the literature have rendered similar findings.[2,5] These studies must be interpreted carefully because volume estimates are often used, and a direct comparison between the office-based and hospital/ASC setting was not always implemented.

It is important to note that the majority of the literature regarding office-based procedures originates from the general surgery, plastics surgery, and dermatology fields. Specific otolaryngology outcomes data and guidelines are limited. Bensoussan and Anderson[6] investigated their single institutional experience with office-based laryngeal procedures to include injection laryngoplasty, Botox for spasmodic dysphonia, laryngeal biopsy, steroid injection, potassium titanyl phosphate (KTP) laser, transnasal esophagostomy, esophageal dilation, and bronchoscopy. Sixteen Canadian laryngologists responded to the survey. The procedures performed in the individual offices were quite varied, as were the instructions to discontinue anticoagulation before the procedure. Sixty percent of the laryngologists premedicated patients with an anxiolytic; the remaining 40% stated that premedication and sedation were never used in their office. Vital signs were routinely documented by only 35.7% of laryngologists. A variety of local anesthetics were used. Most offices did monitor the patient after the procedure for 15 to 30 minutes. With respect to emergency equipment available in the office, 80% had a crash cart and defibrillator, 73% had the ability to treat an allergic reaction, and 67% had the ability to treat laryngospasm. Overall, up to one-third of respondents disclosed a lack of access to medical resources to emergently treat laryngospasm and anaphylactic reactions. Only minor adverse events were reported, including anxiety/patient intolerance, intractable gag/cough, vomiting, vasovagal response, and discomfort/pain. One laryngologist reported a mild, self-limiting episode of laryngospasm. The authors advocate evidence-based practice guidelines dedicated to office-based laryngeal procedures to promote consistent documentation and safety.

The American Academy of Otolaryngology-Head and Neck Surgery/Foundation (AAO-HNS/F) provides position statements with supporting evidence related to office-based procedures such as laryngeal photoangiolytic laser treatment[7] and in-office snoring procedures.[8] Otolaryngologists embarking on office-based procedures are encouraged to remain current on AAO-HNS/F and associated subspecialty society guidelines and positions statements because it remains a dynamic field.

ACCREDITATION AND SAFETY CONSIDERATIONS

It is imperative to recognize specific differences between office-based anesthesia and procedures versus those performed in the hospital and ASC setting. By definition, an office-based surgical procedure is conducted entirely within the doctor's office. As such, an office-based procedure room is exempt from the state-issued certificate of need warranted for an ASC.[9] In fact, most states do not require a license or formal accreditation for the office-based setting. Unlike hospital-based operating rooms and ASCs, office-based surgery centers are not required to report to the government patient safety issues such as transfers to hospitals or deaths.[3,10,11] Therefore, the onus of patient safety and quality care falls directly on the otolaryngologist.

Physicians intending to perform office-based procedures should familiarize themselves with current guidelines. The American Society of Anesthesiologists (ASA) Guidelines for Office-Based Anesthesia specifically state that an office-based procedure room should have a medical director or governing body responsible for policy.[12] The individual must ensure that the facility and personnel are adequate for the types of procedures being conducted. For many offices, this responsibility falls to the practicing otolaryngologist.

The Accreditation Association for Ambulatory Heath Care and the American Association for Accreditation of Ambulatory Surgical Facilities are 2 recognized entities with accreditation power for office-based practices. Although formal accreditation remains voluntary in some states, most require formal accreditation for offices in which anesthesia beyond minimal sedation is used.[9] In addition, government and third-party reimbursement has the potential to be linked to accreditation in a manner similar to The Joint Commission and inpatient services.

The American College of Surgeons (ACS) recognized the disparity in patient safety and guidelines for office-based surgery. In response, they proposed a resolution to the American Medical Association to convene a working group of dedicated specialty societies and state medical associations to identify requirements aimed to optimize patient safety and quality for office-based procedures. Currently, the ACS outlines 10 core patient safety principles for office-base surgery.[13] The most recent list is available at https://www.facs.org/education/patient-education/patient-safety/office-based and incorporates guidelines outlined by the Federation of State Medical Boards. In addition, the ACS advocates facility accreditation by the Joint Commission on Accreditation of Healthcare Organizations, Accreditation Association for Ambulatory Heath Care, American Association for Accreditation of Ambulatory Surgical Facilities, American Osteopathic Association, or by a state-recognized entity.

The Joint Commission on Office-Based Surgery aims to improve patient safety through the publications of national guidelines. The most recent 2019 goals are available online at www.jointcommission.org.[14] In brief, the document states that patients must be identified correctly with at least 2 forms of identification to ensure that each patient receives the correct medication, blood products, and surgery. Medication safety includes labeling all medications to include syringes, cups, and basins. Patient medication lists must be current and well-documented. Hand washing precautions should be implemented per the Centers for Disease Control and Prevention and/or the World Health Organization. Proven guidelines to prevent surgical infection (ie, antibiotic use, surgical site preparation, sterile draping) should be used. Last, surgical site mistakes can be avoided through correct marking of the anatomic surgical site on the patient and a formal surgical time out before commencing surgery.

In addition to these national organizations, various subspecialty societies have established guidelines for office-based procedures. For example, the American Society of Plastic Surgeons mandates that its membership only operates within the context of accredited offices.[9] The American Academy of Dermatology provides guidelines for use of local anesthesia in the office setting to include types of agents, delivery methods, and potential complications.[15] Recommendations include the clear calculation and documentation of local anesthetic used in an attempt to avoid toxicity. Similarly, the Society of American Gastrointestinal Endoscopic Surgeons published office-based endoscopy guidelines to include recommendations related to the physical space, personnel training, patient selection, nil per os (NPO) status, monitoring, periprocedural medications, and documentation.[16] The ASA adopted guidelines for office-based anesthesia emphasizes that the standard anesthetic care in an office surgical suite should be equivalent to that of a hospital or ASC.[11] As discussed above, the AAO-HNS/F has published position statements and guidelines for various in-office procedures.[7,8]

EQUIPMENT AND PROTOCOLS

The ASA recommends monitoring with pulse oximetry, electrocardiogram, blood pressure, capnography, and temperature for all office-based procedures using sedation.[11] Routine checklists implemented in the office setting have successfully decreased complication rates.[17] Emergency protocols are often written and practiced in the office setting to include the management of malignant hyperthermia (MH) crisis, cardiopulmonary emergencies, airway fire, internal and external disasters, and emergency transfer to a hospital. Similarly, a host of checklists are available through the World Health Organization, Association of PeriOperative Registered Nurses, the American Association of Nurse Anesthetists, the Institute for Safety in Office-Based Surgery, ACS, and Society of Ambulatory Anesthesia, as well as other subspecialty societies.[9,11,12,18] Common themes transcend the various guidelines:

- Office facilities should comply with federal, state, and local laws, codes, and regulations.
- The standard of anesthesia care in the office setting should mirror that of the hospital and an ASC.
- At a minimum, office-based procedure rooms should provide oxygen, suction, resuscitation equipment, and emergency medications.
- All equipment should be maintained, tested, and inspected per manufacturer's specifications.
- Offices in which procedures are being conducted should have adequately trained personal (ie, basic life support [BLS], advanced cardiovascular life support [ACLS], and pediatric advance life support) as indicated.

- Offices must have emergency equipment and associated medications to address emergencies to include cardiac events, allergic reactions, laryngospasm, loss of airway, and MH if succinylcholine is being used (**Box 1**).
- The duration and complexity of the procedure should permit patient timely recovery and discharge to home. The decision for discharge falls to the physician and should be well-documented.

PATIENT AND PROCEDURE SELECTION

Patient selection is critical in the decision to perform an office-based procedure. **Box 2** provides a list of poor candidates who would be better served in a hospital setting. A thorough review of the patient's past medical history is imperative and should include active medications, drug and latex allergies, psychological history with emphasis on anxiety, family history of MH, and high-risk conditions such as morbid obesity, obstructive sleep apnea, and a difficulty airway.[9,18] Higher risk patients are often treated in procedure rooms or endoscopy suites at a hospital or ASC where more resources are available for potentially higher acuity cases.[19]

Box 1
Potential in-office otolaryngology procedure room needs beyond surgical equipment

Monitoring
- Noninvasive blood pressure
- Heart rate
- Electrocariograph
- Temperature
- Capnography

Airway supplies
- Supplemental oxygen with regulators (minimum of 2 sources)
- Nasal cannula and face mask
- Oral airways
- Self-inflating bag-mask ventilation device (Ambu bag)
- Laryngoscope (Macintosh and Miller; various sizes)
- Endotracheal tubes and stylets
- Supraglottic airway device (laryngeal mask airway)
- Glidescope
- Suction equipment to include tubing, catheters, and Yankaur suctions

Additional emergency equipment
- Compression board
- Tracheostomy/cricothyrotomy kit
- Charged cardiac defibrillator
- ACLS drugs
- Malignant hyperthermia supplies to include dantrolene (Ryanodex)
- 20% lipid emulsion for local anesthetic systemic toxicity
- Emergency power source

Box 2
Poor surgical candidates for office-based otolaryngology procedures[23]

- Morbid obesity
- Severe obstructive sleep apnea
- Potential for a difficult airway
- High aspiration risk
- Anaphylaxis risk
- Malignant hyperthermia
- History of adverse anesthesia event
- Severe chronic obstructive pulmonary disease
- Seizure disorder
- Recent myocardial infarction
- Recent stroke
- Abnormal bleeding/clotting disorder
- Deep vein thrombosis risk
- Sickle cell disease
- Poorly controlled diabetes mellitus
- Poorly controlled hypertension
- History of substance abuse
- Severe anxiety
- Cognitive inability to cooperate
- Severe craniofacial anomalies/retrognathia/micrognathia
- Significant trismus

Equally important is procedure selection. Technical advances in both surgery and anesthesia allow for procedures with greater complexity and increased duration to transpire in the office setting. However, both variables must be considered thoughtfully when scheduling patients. Increased surgery duration correlates with a higher incidence of postoperative nausea, vomiting, bleeding, pain, and ultimately unplanned hospital admission.[20–22] The American Society of Plastic Surgeons currently recommends that office-based procedures be limited to 6 hours duration and be completed by 3 PM.[23]

Anesthetic needs must also be taken into consideration when deciding on the operative setting. The ASA recognizes 4 levels of sedation (**Fig. 1**).[24] Deep sedation (level III) and general anesthesia (level IV) are identified as less safe in the office setting.[24,25] Additional considerations include expected blood loss and associated need for blood products, anticipated major fluid shifts, and the likelihood of postoperative opioid need.

LOCAL ANESTHETIC OPTIONS

The majority of office-based otolaryngology procedures are performed using local anesthesia alone. Lidocaine is the most common agent for local infiltration. It is a member of the amide family, which also includes articaine, bupivacaine, etidocaine,

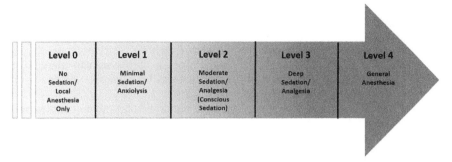

Fig. 1. Continuum of sedation and anesthesia.

mepivacaine, and prilocaine. The maximum lidocaine dose for a healthy adult is 4.5 mg/kg or 300 mg when injected alone. If lidocaine is mixed with the vasoconstrictor epinephrine, this dosage can be increased to 7.0 mg/kg or a total of 500 mg.[15] Local anesthetics in the ester family are recommended for patients with a known lidocaine allergy.[15] This category includes chloroprocaine, procaine, and tetracaine. Needle aspiration should be performed before injection to avoid intravascular administration. The slow infiltration of a warm solution can minimize pain, as can the application of a topical anesthetic at the injection site, the use of a skin-vibrating device, and the addition of sodium bicarbonate.[15]

Local anesthesia can be used to anesthetize the immediate surrounding tissues of the surgical bed or as an injection for regional cutaneous nerve blockade. **Fig. 2** summarizes common local blocks implemented for otolaryngology procedures. Additional areas of local anesthesia infiltration include the larynx via flexible endoscopy or transtracheal injection. In addition, the maxillary nerve can be blocked via infiltration into the greater palatine foreman. The foreman is located adjacent to the second and third maxillary molar, 1 cm toward midline, just anterior to the juncture of the hard and soft palate. Prebending the needle at the 1-cm mark will ensure avoidance of deep injection. The posterior portion of the hard palate, soft tissues surrounding the first bicuspid, and the distribution of the nasopalatine nerve will be anesthetized with this block.

Block	Location	Area Anesthetized
1. Infraorbital Nerve	5–7 mm below rim; Foramen aligns with medial limbus of iris	Lower eyelid; cheek; nasal sidewall; upper lip
2. Mental Nerve	With lower lip retracted, inject lateral to canine	Lower lip; chin
3. Supraorbital Nerve/ Supratrochlear Nerve	Superior edge middle 1/3 of eyebrow	Upper eyelid; forehead
4. Dorsal Nasal Block	Nerve exits along caudal edge, 6–10 mm from midline	Nasal dorsum and tip
5. Zygomaticotemporal	10–12 mm posterior to lateral orbital rim	Lateral canthus; temporal hairline/scalp
6. Zygomaticofacial	Lateral aspect of inferior orbital rim	Mid-cheek
7. Greater Auricular Nerve	6.5 cm below EAC at mid SCM	Lower 1/3 auricle; post-auricular region; tragus extending inferior to mandible
8. Trigeminal Nerve (V3)	Sigmoid notch; 2.5 cm anterior to tragus	Cheek; superior preauricular region; auriculotemporal region

Fig. 2. Common otolaryngology regional nerve blocks. EAC, external auditory canal; SCM, sternocleidomastoid muscle.

Physicians and nurses managing the care of patients undergoing local anesthesia must be well-versed in the signs and symptoms of systemic toxicity.[15,18] Patients may develop central nervous system complaints, including tinnitus, circumoral paresthesia, or a metallic taste. Patients can develop dysarthria, seizures, loss of consciousness, and ultimately respiratory arrest. From a cardiovascular standpoint, local anesthesia toxicity can manifest as hypotension, bradycardia, ventricular arrhythmias, and/or cardiovascular arrest.

Careful calculation and documentation of medication administration coupled with constant patient communication minimizes the risk of toxicity. Lipid emulsion 20% remains the standard of care for local anesthetic systemic toxicity (LAST), regardless of local anesthetic used. The American Society of Regional Anesthesia and Pain Management recommends that offices performing local anesthesia maintain a LAST Rescue Kit[26] composed of:

1. 1 L (total) lipid emulsion 20%
2. Several large syringes and needles for rapid infusion
3. Standard intravenous tubing
4. A printed LAST checklist

A clearly developed protocol for local toxicity should be established in all offices performing patient procedures under local anesthesia. The recommended American Society of Regional Anesthesia checklist is summarized in **Box 3**.[26]

Box 3
American Society of Regional Anesthesia and Pain Management recommended checklist for treatment of LAST

- Call for help

- Call for LAST Rescue Kit (see below)

- Administer lipid emulsion therapy at the first sign of serious toxicity
  - Bolus of 100 mL of lipid emulsion 20% should be rapidly administered over 2 to 3 minutes for patients >70 kg
  - Bolus of 1.5 mL/kg for patients <70 kg
  - Lipid emulsion should not exceed 12 mL/kg total

- Alert nearest cardiopulmonary bypass team if resuscitation is prolonged

- Airway management
  - 100% oxygen administration
  - Avoid hyperventilation
  - Advanced airway device for respiratory depression

- Seizure control
  - Benzodiazepines preferred
  - Avoid large doses of propofol

- Cardiovascular collapse
  - Treat hypotension
  - Treat bradycardia
  - Institute basic life support/ACLS protocols if pulseless

- Prolonged monitoring for 2 to 6 hours is recommended owing to the potential for recurrence of cardiovascular depression

Adapted from Neal JM, Barrington MJ, Fettiplace MR, et al. The Third American Society of Regional Anesthesia and Pain Medicine Practice Advisory on Local Anesthetic Systemic Toxicity: Executive Summary 2017, 2018;43:113–123; with permission.

PROCEDURAL SEDATION

The American College of Emergency Physicians defines procedural sedation as "a technique of administering sedatives or dissociative agents with or without analgesics to induce a state that allows the patient to tolerate unpleasant procedures while maintaining cardiorespiratory function."[27] The goal of procedural sedation and analgesia is to depress the level of consciousness while allowing the patient to maintain independent oxygenation and airway control. **Fig. 1** summarizes the various levels of sedation which are a continuum. Level I is minimal sedation, limited to anxiolysis. Patients maintain the ability to respond to verbal stimuli and there is no impact on airway protection, spontaneous ventilation, or cardiovascular function.[18,27] Level II is moderate sedation with analgesia, often termed conscious sedation. Patients demonstrate purposeful response to verbal and tactile stimuli and airway intervention is not usually required, because patients can maintain adequate spontaneous ventilation. Similarly, cardiovascular function is usually maintained. Level III is deemed deep sedation with analgesia. Patient are able to respond to repeat, painful stimuli (usually not verbal). Airway intervention may be required owing to inadequate spontaneous ventilation, but cardiovascular function is usually still maintained. Last, level IV is general anesthesia, under which patients are unarousable, event to painful stimuli. Spontaneous ventilation is frequently inadequate, warranting airway intervention, and cardiovascular function may be impaired.

It is important to note that monitored anesthesia care does not fit directly into the continuum pictured in **Fig. 1** because it does not describe a specific level of sedation, but rather a service in which an anesthesiologist has been requested to participate in the care of a patient undergoing an office-based procedure.[27] In addition, it is impossible to predict an individual patient's response to the various levels of sedation along the continuum. Therefore, otolaryngologists performing office-based sedation must be prepared to rescue a patient with appropriate airway and advanced life support in the event that a deeper level of sedation is encountered.[27]

A broad host of medications are available for procedural sedation. Opioids (morphine, fentanyl, and remifentanil) provide analgesia with possible sedation. Naloxone should be readily available in the office for acute reversal. Benzodiazepines such as diazepam, midazolam, and lorazepam produce anxiolysis, sedation, and amnesia, but they do not provide analgesic properties. Anesthesia induction medications including barbiturates have fallen out of favor owing to agents such as propofol and ketamine, which are easier to titrate. Last, inhaled anesthetics include nitrous oxide, isoflurane, desflurane, sevoflurane, and halothane. It is the physician's responsibility to have a clear understanding of dosage, pharmacokinetics, and side effects, which is beyond the scope of this article.

A thorough history and physical examination must be conducted before administering sedation. Patients with a history of anesthesia/sedation complications, obstructive sleep apnea, stridor/snoring, and chromosomal abnormality such as trisomy 21 are considered poor candidates for in-office sedation. Additional contraindications include morbid obesity, limited neck extension, tracheal deviation, trismus, and dysmorphic facial features such as Pierre-Robin syndrome and micrognathia/retorgnathia.[27]

OFFICE-BASED COMPLICATIONS AND EMERGENCIES

Any office-based procedure using local anesthesia or sedation has the potential for an allergic reaction or toxicity. As outlined above, a LAST rescue kit[26] with a written protocol is essential for all offices in which local anesthesia is being administered, even in the absence of sedation (level 0). **Box 1** summarizes additional equipment necessary for office-based procedures in which sedation is being administered, regardless of level. Additionally, the American Association of Nurse Anesthetists recommends written policies for ACLS algorithms and resuscitation plans, latex allergy, and pediatric drug dosages if applicable.[18] Similar emergency protocols should be written to address environmental emergencies such as chemical spills, fire, building evacuation, and bomb threat.

MH is a rare but potentially fatal familial, skeletal muscle syndrome in which a hypermetabolic reaction is triggered by volatile anesthetic gases or depolarizing muscle relaxants such as succinylcholine.[28] Early recognition is imperative. Early clinical signs include an acute increase in end-tidal CO_2 levels, tachycardia and other cardiac arrhythmias, muscle rigidity to include trismus, hypoxia, profuse sweating, unstable arterial pressures, metabolic–respiratory acidosis, and skin mottling.[29,30] If timely intervention is not administered, patients can develop myoglobinurea and acute renal failure, cardiovascular failure, hyperkalemia, hyperthermia, hypotension, and rhabdomyolysis.[29,30]

Early recognition and rapid administration of dantrolene directly correlates with survival.[31] Upon recognition of MH, the inciting agent must be discontinued and eliminated with the placement of charcoal filters on the anesthesia circuit; 100% oxygen should be administered.[18] The priority is then cooling and stabilization for transfer to a hospital intensive care unit setting. The American Association of Nurse Anesthetists recommends a dedicated MH emergency cart to include dantrolene, sterile water for injection, sodium bicarbonate, dextrose 50%, calcium chloride 10%, 100 U/mL regular insulin, 2% lidocaine for injection, and refrigerated cold saline solution (3000 mL minimum).[18]

All otolaryngologists performing office-based procedures should have a hospital agreement and transfer policy in the rare event that an emergency occurs. The Federation of State Medical Boards strongly encourages reporting of adverse events, hospital transfers, patient deaths within 30 days of the office-based procedure, observation for more than 24 hours, and unscheduled readmission within 72 hours of the procedure.[1] This reporting mechanism is usually via a designated state agency, confidential, and intended for quality improvement purposes. An internal peer-review process provides an additional quality improvement opportunity.

SUMMARY

A host of otolaryngology procedures lend themselves to the office-based setting. Although regulations for office-based surgeries are not as stringent as traditional hospital operating rooms and ASCs, it is imperative for the physician to be well-versed in state and society regulations, as well as relevant practice guidelines. To deliver safe and effective care, the office must have adequate equipment, medications, and written procedures to address all emergencies from allergic reactions and systemic toxicity from local anesthesia to MH. Ultimately, the office-based procedure setting must have same standards to include emergency equipment, trained personal, and safety measures as that provided in a hospital-based setting and ASCs.

REFERENCES

1. Report of the special committee on outpatient (office-based) surgery. Federation of State Medical Boards. Available at: http://www.fsmb.org/advocacy/policies. Accessed July 1, 2018.

2. Hancox JG, Venkat AP, Coldiron B, et al. The safety of office-based surgery: review of recent literature from several disciplines. Arch Dermatol 2004;140: 1379–82.

3. Vila H Jr, Soto R, Cantor AB, et al. Comparative outcomes analysis of procedures performed in physician offices and ambulatory surgery centers. Arch Surg 2003; 138:991–5.

4. Starling J 3rd, Thosani MK, Coldiron BM. Determining the safety of office-based surgery: what 10 years of Florida data and 6 years of Alabama data reveal. Dermatol Surg 2012;38(2):171–7.

5. Kurrek MM, Twersky RS. Office-based anesthesia. Can J Anaesth 2010;57: 353–67.

6. Bensoussan Y, Anderson J. In-office laryngeal procedures (IOLP) in Canada: current safety practices and procedural care. J Otolaryngol Head Neck Surg 2018; 47:23–9.

7. Position statement: in-office photoangiolytic laser treatment of laryngeal pathology. American Academy of Otolaryngology-Head & Neck Surgery/Foundation. Available at: https://www.entnet.org//content/office-photoangiolytic-laser-treatment-laryngeal-pathology. Accessed July 1, 2018.

8. Treatment options for adults with snoring. American Academy of Otolaryngology-Head & Neck Surgery/Foundation. Available at: https://www.entnet.org//content/treatment-options-adults-snoring. Accessed July 1, 2018.

9. Hausman LM. Office-based otolaryngology. In: Levine AI, Govindaraj S, DeMaria Jr S, editors. Anesthesiology and otolaryngology. New York: Springer; 2013. p. 365–71.

10. Cato D. Explaining differences in outpatient surgery. Fort Myers (FL): News-Press; 2018. Available at: https://www.news-press.com/story/opinion/contributors/2018/03/16/explaining-differences-outpatient-surgery/421023002/. Accessed July 1, 2018.

11. Shapiro FE, Punwani N, Rosenberg NM, et al. Office-based anesthesia: safety and outcomes. Anesth Analg 2014;119:276–85.

12. Guidelines for office-based anesthesia. Schaumburg (IL): American Society of Anesthesiologists Ambulatory Surgery Care Committee; 2009. Available at: http://www.asahq.org/quality-and-practice-management/standards-guidelines-and-related-resources/guidelines-for-office-based-anesthesia. Accessed July 1, 2018.

13. Patient safety principles of office-based surgery. American College of Surgeons. Available at: https://www.facs.org/education/patient-education/patient-safety/office-based surgery. Accessed July 1, 2018.

14. 2018 Office-based surgery national patient safety goals. The Joint Commission Accreditation Office Based Surgery. Available at: https://www.jointcommission.org/obs_2017_npsgs/. Accessed July 1,2018.

15. Kouba DJ, LoPiccolo MC, Alam M, et al. Guidelines for use of local anesthesia in office- based dermatological surgery. J Am Acad Dermatol 2016;74:1201–19.

16. Heneghan S, Myers J, Fanelii R, et al. Society of American Gastrointestinal Endoscopic Surgeons (SAGES) guidelines for office endoscopic services. Surg Endosc 2009;23:1125–9.

17. Rosenberg NM, Urman RD, Gallager S, et al. Effect of an office-based surgical safety system on patient outcomes. Eplasty 2012;12:e59.

18. Standard for office based anesthesia practice. American Association of Nurse Anesthetists. Available at: https://www.aana.com/patients/office-based-anesthesia. Accessed July 1, 2018.

19. Collins TR. Adding Office-based laryngeal procedures to your practice can benefit patients. ENT Today 2015.
20. Mingus ML, Bodian CA, Bradford CN, et al. Prolonged surgery increases the likelihood of admission of schedule ambulatory surgery patients. J Clin Anesth 1997; 9:446–50.
21. Fortier J, Chung F, Su J. Unanticipated admission after ambulatory surgery- a prospective study. Can J Anaesth 1998;45:612–9.
22. Gold BS, Kitz DS, Lecky JH, et al. Unanticipated admission to the hospital following ambulatory surgery. JAMA 1989;262:3008–10.
23. Iverson RE, ASPS Task Force on Patient Safety in Office-Based Surgery Facilities. Patient safety in office-based surgery facilities: I. Procedures in the office-based surgery setting. Plast Reconstr Surg 2002;110:1337–42.
24. Continuum of depth of sedation: definition of general anesthesia and levels of sedation. American Society of Anesthesia. Available at: http://www.asahq.org/quality-and-practice-management/standards-guidelines-and-related-resources/continuum-of-depth-of-sedation-definition-of-general-anesthesia-and-levels-of-sedation-analgesia. Accessed July 1, 2018.
25. Hausman LM, Rosenblatt M. Office-based anesthesia. In: Barash PG, editor. Clinical anesthesia, vol. 61, 7th edition. Philadelphia: Lippincott Williams & Wilkins; 2013. p. 983.
26. Checklist for treatment of local anesthetic systemic toxicity (LAST). American Society of Regional Anesthesia and Pain Mediation. Available at: https://www.asra.com/advisory-guidelines/article/3/checklist-for-treatment-of-local-anesthetic-systemic-toxicity. Accessed July 1, 2018.
27. Practice guidelines for moderate procedural sedation and analgesia 2018: a report by the American Society of Anesthesiologists Task Force on Moderate Procedural Sedation and Analgesia, the American Association of Oral and Maxillofacial Surgeons, American College of Radiology, American Dental Association, American Society of Dentist Anesthesiologists, and Society of Interventional Radiology. Anesthesiology 2018;128:437–80.
28. Gurunluoglu R, Swanson JA, Haeck PC, ASPS Patient Safety Committee. Evidence-based patient safety advisory: malignant hyperthermia. Plast Reconstr Surg 2009;124:68S–81S.
29. Seifert PC, Wahr JA, Pace M, et al. Crisis management of malignant hyperthermia in the OR. AORN J 2014;100:189–202.e1.
30. Schneiderbanger D, Johannsen S, Roewer N, et al. Management of malignant hyperthermia: diagnosis and treatment. Ther Clin Risk Manag 2014;10:355–62.
31. Glahn KP, Ellis FR, Halsall PJ, et al. Recognizing and managing a malignant hyperthermia crisis: guidelines from the European Malignant Hyperthermia Group. Br J Anaesth 2010;105:417–20.

Reprocessing Flexible Endoscopes in the Otolaryngology Clinic

Melissa A. Pynnonen, MD, MSc[a],*, John Whelan, BSN, RN[b]

KEYWORDS

- Disinfection • Sterilization • Reprocess • Instructions for use
- Spaulding Classification • Endoscope • Reusable medical device

KEY POINTS

- Reprocessing a flexible endoscope is a complex multistep process. Attention to detail is essential for patient safety.
- Physicians need to empower their staff to function as guardians and advocates for best practices in endoscope reprocessing.
- Current best practice standards and guidelines for flexible endoscope reprocessing in the United States have been led by the Society of Gastroenterology Nurses and Associates, Inc (SGNA), the Association for the Advancement of Medical Instrumentation (AAMI), Association of periOperative Registered Nurses (AORN), American Society for Gastrointestinal Endoscopy (ASGE), and Multisociety Guideline (MSG).

INTRODUCTION

Any reusable medical device has the potential to transmit infection between patients.[1-5] In recent years, multiple examples of infection and deaths linked to reusable medical devices have highlighted the inherent risks with improper and/or incomplete cleaning and disinfection. For 8 of the last 10 years ECRI (formerly the "Emergency Care Research Institute") has identified risk of infection from inadequate endoscope reprocessing as one of the top 10 health hazards in the United States.[6]

From a cleaning and disinfection perspective, channeled flexible endoscopes are the most complex medical devices to reprocess for reuse. Technological advancements have made endoscopic examinations and interventions commonplace. However, the consistent use of best practices for device cleaning and disinfection have not kept pace with device design; and patients have been put at risk.

Disclosure Statement: The authors have nothing to disclose.
[a] University of Michigan, 1904 Taubman Center, 1500 East Medical Center Drive, Ann Arbor, MI 48109-5312, USA; [b] 2033 Norfolk Street, Ann Arbor, MI 48103, USA
* Corresponding author.
E-mail address: pynnonen@med.umich.edu

This article focuses on important aspects and current best practices for flexible endoscope cleaning and high-level disinfection. The basic principles and steps of these detailed processes are also relevant to reprocessing any other reusable instrument in the outpatient clinic.

HISTORY OF ENDOSCOPIC PROCEDURES

Flexible endoscopes first became available in the 1950s,[7–9] initially for examination of the stomach and duodenum, and later for examination of the biliary system[10] and colon.[11,12] Subsequent improvements in light source design and material pliability—combined with multichannel design—enabled endoscopic intervention as well as examination. For example, one channel allowed suction, while a separate channel provided the passage of an instrument, such as for biopsy or laser treatment.

The continued evolution of technological and design improvements now permits thousands of gastrointestinal (GI) endoscopies, laryngoscopies, nasal endoscopies, cystoscopies, and hysteroscopies to be performed every year. Such advancements have allowed endoscopic procedures to transition from the operating room to clinic settings, as well as from hospital to outpatient settings. Unfortunately, attention to, and meticulous implementation of, best practices for cleaning and disinfection of endoscopes have not kept pace with the technical advances.

Implementation of best practices for flexible endoscopic reprocessing requires time commitment and fastidious attention to detail. Unfortunately, observational studies have demonstrated pervasive lapses in technique. In 1 study of manual cleaning followed by automated reprocessing, the steps were performed correctly only 1.4% of the time, whereas automated cleaning and automated reprocessing was better, but not perfect, being done correctly 75% of the time (**Box 1**).[13]

INFECTION PREVENTION

The Spaulding Classification describes the appropriate level of disinfection for medical devices according to their intended use.[14,15] According to the Spaulding Classification, items that contact intact skin (blood pressure cuffs, office furniture, stethoscopes) are classified as "non-critical" devices and require low- or intermediate-level disinfection, for example, surface disinfectant wipes. Items that contact mucous membranes or non-intact skin (flexible or rigid endoscopes, vaginal speculae) are classified as "semi-critical" devices and require high-level disinfection (HLD) or sterilization. Items that penetrate mucosal surfaces (biopsy forceps), or enter the vascular system (vascular catheters) or sterile body cavities (surgical forceps, retractors) require sterilization (**Fig. 1** and **Table 1**).

High-level disinfection refers to elimination of all viable microorganisms except for a small number of spores.[16] Common methods of achieving HLD in the United States include orthophthaldehyde (OPA), glutaraldehyde, peracetic acid, 2% accelerated hydrogen peroxide, or activated H_2O_2 mist (Trophon: Nanosonics Limited, Lane Cove, NSW, Australia).

Sterilization refers to complete elimination of all forms of viable microorganisms including spores. Common methods of sterilization include steam or gas processes. In a clinic setting, this would involve use of an autoclave (steam sterilization). The Spaulding Classification in conjunction with the device manufacturer's instructions for use (IFU) determine the minimal level of disinfection for each device.[1,16,17]

Box 1
Environmental tour checklist for endoscopic reprocessing areas

Physical space:
- Is the area sized appropriately in relation to the volume of equipment processed?
- Do staff put on personal protective equipment (PPE) before entering the area?
- Are staff wearing suitable PPE?
  Is there sufficient work space?
- Are cleaning supplies, storage areas, and other critical items clearly labeled?
- Is there an appropriate hand washing station?
- Is there an appropriate eyewash station?
- Are "dirty" areas physical separate from "clean" ones?
- Are there suitable storage areas for cleaned endoscopes? On visual inspection, do these areas look clean, free of debris, and dry?
- If a cabinet serves as storage, does the cabinet have doors?
- Are endoscope storage containers dry and located off the ground?
- What is the route from the processor to the cabinet? (The route should not cross through the soiled processing area.)

Ventilation:
- Is there negative air pressure to surrounding areas?
- Are air exchange rates and filtration efficiencies appropriate? Is there a minimum of 10 exchanges per hour, with at least 2 being with fresh, outside air?
- Is exhaust vented directly outside?

Documentation and training:
- Are staff aware of the number of endoscopes in the department?
- Does staff know how frequently these are maintained and how that maintenance occurs?
- When staff members are questioned, can they show where evidence-based practices and guidelines are located?
- When staff are asked about their training, does it appear they were trained using the guidelines?
- Are staff given periodic refresher training?

© 2014 The Joint Commission. Joint Commission Online. April 8, 2014. Used with permission. Available at: https://www.jointcomission.org/assets/1/23/jconline_April_9_14.pdf. Accessed March 7, 2019.

PAST PRACTICES AND RECENT CONCERNS

Historically, providers have had a general lack of understanding about the level of contamination and risk of exposure to contagion with reusable medical devices. The AIDS crisis triggered widespread use of personal protective equipment (PPE) in health care (gloves, gowns, masks) and, coincidentally, providers gradually became aware of the inherent risks with reusable devices. However, to this date we remain unaware of the magnitude of the problem because "reprocessing lapses are rarely reported in medical journals leading to the false conclusion that reprocessing lapses are rare."[18,19]

Endoscopic sheaths were developed in an attempt to avoid contamination of the endoscope itself. The disposable sheath covered the fiberoptic tube, with the mistaken belief that it prevented contamination and avoided the need to disinfect the endoscope between uses.[20–22] Providers believed that changing the sheath was all that was required. However, sheaths do not protect the eyepiece or control head, and those sites remain at risk of contamination and sheaths can fail, analogous to a condom. Consequently, the scope still requires HLD to decontaminate these sites. Also, manufacturers' IFUs for current-generation flexible endoscopes prescribe full immersion HLD, or sterilization of the entire device after each use.

Recently, there is increased awareness of the internal damage and residual bio-burden risk for medical devices (including endoscopes).[23] In addition, the appearance

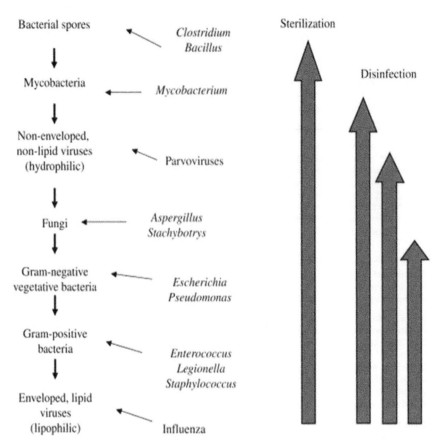

Fig. 1. Relative resistance of typical microorganisms according to level of disinfection or sterilization. (*From* McDonnell G, Burke P. Disinfection: is it time to reconsider Spaulding? J Hosp Infect 2011;78(3):164; with permission.)

of drug-resistant bacteria, such as carbapenem-resistant Enterobacteriaceae—which has a high mortality rate and for which there is limited or no treatment—further emphasizes the need for adequate manual cleaning and inspection as stringent standard parts of reprocessing.[24]

Table 1
Spaulding classification

Patient Contact	Classification	Examples	Disinfection Required
Intact skin	Non-critical	Office furniture, blood pressure cuff, tuning fork, otoscope	Low-level disinfection
Mucous membranes	Semi-critical	Laryngeal mirrors, endoscopes	High-level disinfection
Sterile sites in the body	Critical	Tissue forceps, hemostats, implants,	Sterilization

Adapted from McDonnell G. When disinfectants may not meet our expectations. Healthcare Purchasing News 2014:68; with permission. Available at: https://www.hpnonline.com/inside/2014-06/June2014.html. Accessed March 7, 2019.

Transport between use, reprocessing, storage, and back to the point-of-use poses additional risk for endoscope and environmental contamination. Not too many years ago, some providers would use the original manufacturer's carrying case for transport of both clean and contaminated endoscopes—without ever considering the carrying case as contaminated. The use of pillow cases or patient belonging bags for transport were also not unheard of. Current best practice dictates lidded solid container transport—either reusable (disinfected between uses) or disposable.

The medical device industry designed sophisticated reusable flexible endoscopes at a speed that outpaced the health care industry's ability to develop reprocessing safety measures. In recent years, the news media and regulatory and accrediting agencies have written more about reprocessing lapses for GI endoscopes than any other type of endoscope; yet any flexible endoscope poses risk if not reprocessed correctly and completely. In 2013, patients were exposed to multidrug-resistant bacteria from duodenoscopes—this tragedy occurred despite the fact that the duodenoscopes had reportedly been reprocessed according to the manufacturer's IFU.[25,26]

As a result of such experiences, GI professional societies in conjunction with US standards (Association for the Advancement of Medical Instrumentation [AAMI], Centers for Disease Control and Prevention, U.S. Food and Drug Administration) accreditation (The Joint Commission [TJC]) and regulatory agencies (U.S. Food and Drug Administration) have increasingly redefined and emphasized best practices for reprocessing flexible endoscopes of any kind. For years, the SGNA[1] and the MSG[5] set the bar for flexible endoscope reprocessing standards. In recent years, the addition of AAMI's Standard 91 has further defined expected practices.[2]

HIGH-LEVEL DISINFECTION VERSUS STERILIZATION

Currently, not all flexible endoscopes are designed to be sterilized. The lengths and overall size of some endoscopes, their material construction, and the presence of interior channels and surfaces can preclude use of, or complete and effective penetration for, gas plasma or steam sterilization methods. Ethylene oxide sterilization is not readily available, is costly, and is highly regulated in the United States.[27] For these reasons liquid chemical HLD remains the common reprocessing endpoint for flexible endoscopes.

The use and reprocessing for non-channeled, less-complex endoscopes (eg, laryngoscopes, nasal endoscopes) also pose risk. Any incomplete cleaning and/or disinfection, as well as scope damage, can result in transmission of infection.

Rigid endoscopes and instruments may be sterilized by various methods: steam under pressure (autoclave), low temperature, hydrogen peroxide gas plasma (STERRAD), or ethylene oxide gas. In response to recent infection transmissions linked to flexible endoscopes, some experts have suggested that we should revise the Spaulding Classification by moving beyond HLD and toward sterilization of all flexible endoscopes.[28] Currently, not all flexible endoscopes can be sterilized. Some sterilization methods can damage scopes. Sterilization infrastructure and capacity are not commonly available within clinic and ambulatory care settings. Device manufacturers are currently developing more options for disposable or sterilizable endoscopes, whereas equipment manufacturers strive to create low-temperature sterilization methods that are readily available and applicable to a wider range of flexible endoscopes.

Importantly, moving from HLD to sterilization does not abdicate the need for emphasis on adequate manual cleaning before disinfection. A device cannot be effectively disinfected or sterilized if it is not completely clean.

MANUAL CLEANING BEFORE DISINFECTION

Recent years have seen increased focus on the need for monitoring and validating the manual cleaning for flexible endoscopes. Experts agree on manual cleaning as the most crucial step in reprocessing. The multiple steps of manual cleaning are necessary to mechanically remove bioburden ("wash the dishes") and prevent subsequent biofilm formation (see later discussion current best practice for reprocessing flexible endoscopes). Post cleaning verification methods—such as adenosine triphosphate testing—can be used at the end of manual cleaning and before the scope proceeds to disinfection/sterilization.[29] This can serve as a benchmark for whether cleaning was adequate.

MANUAL AND AUTOMATED REPROCESSING

Endoscopes may be reprocessed by either manual or automated methods, this is an individual choice for each clinic based on patient volume, staffing resources, and the considerable expense of automated endoscope reprocessors (AERs). Most otolaryngology clinics use a manual process. The completely manual process includes: validating effectiveness and temperature for the disinfectant soak bath with each use, donning and doffing PPE, flushing channels with syringes, monitoring the disinfectant soak time, manual rinsing/flushing with water, then alcohol, and documenting the cycle detail. Automated endoscope reprocessors replace and standardize many if not all of the labor-intensive manual steps. Some AERs provide automated cycles for detergent cleaning and rinsing as well. From process effectiveness and quality control perspectives, automated processes are seen to limit risks because of human error. In recent years, automated leak testing, flushing devices, and forced air drying have added options to limit human error through systematic processes.

CHEMICAL HIGH-LEVEL DISINFECTION PROCESSES

Glutaraldehyde (Cidex, Sonacide, Sporicidin, Hospex, Omnicide, Metricide, Rapicide, and Wavicide) was commonly used worldwide for endoscope disinfection because it was often the least expensive disinfectant, and did not damage endoscopes. However, because of safety and environmental concerns the agent has been banned in some locations.[30] In the United States there is increasing interest in using alternative chemical methods.

Orthophthaldehyde is safe for endoscopes and is a common disinfectant for reprocessing in the United States. However, anaphylactic reactions have occurred in some patients undergoing urologic procedures; as a result cystoscopes and urologic devices are typically not reprocessed in OPA.[31]

Peracetic acid (Rapicide PA) is a chemical disinfectant used in automated reprocessing. It has served as a valid alternative for glutaraldehyde (safety concerns) and OPA (for urologic devices).

Lastly, 2% accelerated hydrogen peroxide (Revital-Ox RESERT) is a high-level disinfectant used in manual and automated reprocessing. It has a shorter soak time (8 minutes for Revital-Ox RESERT compared with 12 or 30 minutes for OPA and glutaraldehyde, respectively). RESERT is currently not validated for use by all endoscope manufacturers and/or AER manufacturers.[32]

CURRENT BEST PRACTICE FOR REPROCESSING FLEXIBLE ENDOSCOPES

Currently, the best practice for HLD is outlined by 9 basic steps of reprocessing outlined below.[1,33] In addition, these steps should be supplemented with additional brand- and/or model-specific measures provided by each manufacturer's IFU. It is important to note that endoscope reprocessing exposes the medical assistant to harmful chemicals and body fluids. Thus, proper PPE must be worn as prescribed by Occupational Safety and Health Administration standards.[34]

Large health care institutions typically have infection control staff with sufficient expertise to educate and train staff in best practices for HLD. However, in other settings training resources may be scarce. Formal training and certification is available and can provide a foundational understanding of the relevant scientific principles, and develop skills and assess competency for staff responsible for HLD. Examples of HLD training programs include:

- Certified Endoscope Reprocessor certification—https://www.iahcsmm.org/certification-menu/cer-certification.html
- Flexible Endoscope Reprocessor (GI Scope) Certification Exam (C.F.E.R.)—http://www.sterileprocessing.org/gi.htm
- SGNA Infection Prevention Champions program—https://www.sgna.org/Practice/Infection-Prevention

Step 1 Pre-cleaning

Pre-cleaning occurs before the endoscope leaves the patient care area. Pre-cleaning involves wiping down the endoscope to remove visible debris as well as flushing or suctioning through any channels. Enzymatic detergent is often used to begin the breakdown of bioburden. The pre-cleaning objectives are to prevent bioburden from drying and adhering to the device, and to prevent biofilm formation. Both substances are more difficult to remove in subsequent steps— thereby lessening the efficacy of the overall decontamination process (whether that is HLD or sterilization). Research has shown the microbial load is reduced significantly with complete pre-cleaning before the material has a chance to dry.[13,35–38] Delayed reprocessing also increases the risk of ineffective decontamination. The endoscope should then be transported without delay—to a dedicated soiled reprocessing room—in a rigid container with a lid. The container should be clearly marked "biohazard." Reusable transport containers for dirty scopes must be wiped down with an approved low-level disinfectant after each soiled transport.

Step 2. Leak Testing

The need for leak testing of a particular model of flexible endoscope is determined by the manufacturer's IFU. Most current-generation flexible endoscopes do require leak testing; and this occurs each time the scope is reprocessed—at the beginning of the process. A leak may or may not be visible and it can occur anywhere inside or outside the scope. If a leak is present, it can allow fluid as well as bioburden to enter the interior of the scope, which can result in extensive damage, as well as risk to the next patient. If a leak is present, the scope must be sent for repair. It is important to note that a scope still requires cleaning and disinfection before sending for repair; but prescribed alternate steps are taken to protect the scope from further damage during reprocessing.

Step 3. Manual Cleaning

Manual cleaning is a critically important step of scope reprocessing. The scope cannot be cleaned while detachable parts are still attached to the scope. All parts (ie, buttons, caps, adapters) should have been removed for leak testing. Next the scope is submerged in enzymatic detergent. Although submerged, all surfaces of the scope are wiped down with a lint-free cloth or sponge; and all control knobs, ports, and channels are cleaned with unique soft brushes to remove particulate debris which, if retained, will allow for biofilm development and hamper HLD. Channels are flushed and/or suctioned in the amounts and for the length of time prescribed by the IFU.

Step 4. Rinse after Cleaning

The endoscope is completely rinsed and any channels flushed with clean water to remove enzymatic detergent and any residual debris. The endoscope is then dried—to limit dilution of disinfectant in the manual process.

Step 5. Visual Inspection

Careful visual inspection is a purposeful "timeout" at this stage to identify retained debris or any indication of incomplete cleaning. If needed, the scope is manually re-cleaned and re-inspected.

Step 6. High-Level Disinfection

High-level disinfection may be manual or automated. Automated disinfection, using an AER is more common for GI and urologic endoscopes, which are often channeled scopes and, therefore, more challenging to reprocess. Manual reprocessing is the most common HLD method in the outpatient otolaryngology clinic. Manual HLD is accomplished by completely submersing the scope in disinfectant solution. The size of the container must be large enough to avoid excessive coiling. Before HLD for each endoscope the medical assistant must test the concentration of the HLD solution to ensure it meets the minimum effective concentration. The medical assistant must also check and document the temperature of the disinfectant to ensure it is at minimum requirements. All channels must be flushed with disinfectant to ensure there are no air bubbles trapped in the channels that will prevent contact between the disinfectant and the interior walls of the channel. The endoscope must soak in the solution for the time indicated in the disinfectant manufacturer's IFU and the time should be measured with a timing device. The scope should not sit in the solution for an excessive period of time as this can damage the scope, cause surface staining, and require additional rinsing to safely remove excess product from the instrument before patient use.

Step 7. Rinse after High-Level Disinfection

Complete rinsing is necessary to remove residual disinfectant solution and prevent harmful exposure to the patient or provider. Fresh clean water is often used to rinse the exterior and flush all channels, although some IFUs call for a sterile water rinse. Each disinfectant has a specific rinsing protocol. As an example, one brand of OPA disinfectant calls for 3 rinses of 9 L each.

Step 8. Drying

Current best practice calls for drying all channels with forced air to remove residual moisture and lessen the risk of subsequent contamination through growth of residual microorganisms.[39] External surfaces are dried with a lint-free cloth. To speed the drying time, endoscopes can also be wiped down with a gauze soaked in 70% isopropyl alcohol, if prescribed in the IFU. Before transporting the endoscope to storage or a patient care site a label is affixed to the scope as a visual cue indicating that the endoscope has completed the HLD process.[40] At our institution the visual cue is green and labeled with the HLD process date and expiration date (see storage). Following HLD, endoscopes should be transported in a clean rigid container covered with a lid.

Step 9. Storage

Endoscopes must be stored in a manner to prevent contamination from moisture, dust, or contact. Flexible endoscopes are typically stored vertically in a cabinet that allows each endoscope to hang freely without risk of being jostled and damaged. The cabinet doors are kept closed except when in use, and the cabinet is labeled "High-level disinfected. Patient ready." If a flexible endoscope is not used before a determined expiration date, it should be reprocessed before use. The duration of safe hang time is currently unknown. Professional societies and standards vary in their recommendations of "hang time"—how long the HLD scope can remain unused before reprocessing is required. Current best practice is for each practice or health care institution to conduct an individualized risk assessment to determine the length of time before reprocessing is required again.[5] This expiration date does not apply to flexible endoscopes that have been sterilized.

PEARLS FOR OFFICE-BASED HIGH-LEVEL DISINFECTION PROCESSING IN THE OFFICE

1. Become familiar with published best practices for endoscope reprocessing
   a. TJC BoosterPak[16]
   b. Society of Gastroenterology Nurses and Associates, Inc (SGNA)[1]
   c. Association for the Advancement of Medical Instrumentation (AAMI)[2]
   d. Association of periOperative Registered Nurses (AORN)[3]
   e. American Society for Gastrointestinal Endoscopy (ASGE)[4]
   f. Multisociety Guidelines[5]
2. Make sure all providers and clinic staff understand what IFUs are, understand where they are stored in your clinic for reference, and understand that IFUs are not optional.
3. Spend time with your medical assistants and shadow them as they perform tasks of endoscope reprocessing. Observing the HLD process and discussing challenges of the work flow is the most authentic method to identify practice gaps compared with current standards. Insufficient staffing is a prominent challenge in most clinics. The processes for HLD have become progressively more time consuming. If a medical assistant is trying to manage clinic flow while simultaneously being responsible for endoscope reprocessing the medical assistant may feel rushed—resulting in errors and placing patients at risk.
4. Engage your staff in the conversation, emphasizing the need, and empowering them to take ownership for implementing HLD Best Practices in your clinic. Encourage open and process-oriented dialogue focused on preventing misses and near misses.
5. Identify a staff member in your practice who will serve as a champion for HLD processing. This person should be a member of the health care team, as opposed to a member of the clerical staff. At our institution this is typically a lead medical assistant.
6. Develop distinct expectations, processes, and responsibilities—to both empower the HLD champion, as well as to ensure the practice has adequate staff and resources to implement HLD best practice on a daily basis.
7. Hold the practice manager responsible for adequately enabling and empowering any staff who perform reprocessing. Ultimately, management is responsible and

managers are expected to understand the processes performed by the staff they supervise.[16]

8. Develop written standard operating procedures for all reprocessing steps—from pre-cleaning at point-of-use, through reprocessing, to storage. Please see Appendix 1 in the Preface of this issue, by Drs. Pynnonen and Schmalbach, for an example.

9. Establish processes to monitor staff adherence.

10. Staff are expected to have written proof of training and competency on a recurring basis.[16] Please see Appendix 2 in the Preface of this issue, by Drs. Pynnonen and Schmalbach, for an example.

11. Consider investing in your HLD staff by enrolling them in a reprocessing certification program.

SUMMARY

"Flexible endoscope reprocessing has been shown to have a narrow margin of safety. Any slight deviation from the recommended reprocessing protocol can lead to the survival of microorganisms and an increased risk of infection."[40,41] Medical staff adequately educated and empowered to take responsibility for HLD in your practice is your best (and ultimately your last) line of defense. Each clinic must perform a gap analysis and risk assessment considering evidence-based practices and guidelines.[16] As flexible endoscopes and reusable devices have evolved, so has the complexity in reprocessing. Reprocessing standards continue to evolve as well. It will take team effort in your clinic setting to keep abreast of this changing landscape and insure the best outcome for your patients.

ACKNOWLEDGMENTS

Sarah Boyer, MA Lead Specialist and Michigan Medicine Department of Infection Prevention and Epidemiology.

REFERENCES

1. Herrin A, Loyola M, Bocian S, et al. Standards of infection prevention in reprocessing flexible gastrointestinal endoscopes. Gastroenterol Nurs 2016;39(5):404–18.

2. Association for the Advancement of Medical Instrumentation. Flexible and semi-rigid endoscope processing in health care facilities. Arlington (VA): Association for the Advancement of Medical Instrumentation; 2015.

3. AORN. AORN guidelines for perioperative practice 2018. Denver (CO): AORN; 2018.

4. ASGE. Homepage for the American Society Gastrointestinal Education (ASGE) with educational resources and clinical practice guidelines. Available at: https://www.asge.org/search-results?TypeFacet=PracticeGuidelines&keywords=reprocessing. Accessed August 8, 2018.

5. Petersen BT, Cohen J, Hambrick RD, et al. Multisociety guideline on reprocessing flexible GI endoscopes: 2016 update. Gastrointest Endosc 2017;85(2):282–94.e1.

6. Executive brief: top 10 health technology hazards for 2018. Available at: https://www.ecri.org/Resources/Whitepapers_and_reports/Haz_18.pdf. Accessed March 7, 2019.

7. Hirschowitz BI. Endoscopic examination of the stomach and duodenal cap with the fiberscope. Lancet 1961;1(7186):1074–8.

8. Hirschowitz BI. A personal history of the fiberscope. Gastroenterology 1979; 76(4):864–9.

9. Lau WY, Leow CK, Li AK. History of endoscopic and laparoscopic surgery. World J Surg 1997;21(4):444–53.
10. Oi I. Fiberduodenoscopy and endoscopic pancreatocholangiography. Gastrointest Endosc 1970;17(2):59–62.
11. Wolff WI. Colonoscopy: history and development. Am J Gastroenterol 1989;84(9): 1017–25.
12. Overholt BF. Flexible fiberoptic sigmoidoscopes. CA Cancer J Clin 1969;19(2):81–4.
13. Ofstead CL, Wetzler HP, Snyder AK, et al. Endoscope reprocessing methods: a prospective study on the impact of human factors and automation. Gastroenterol Nurs 2010;33(4):304–11.
14. Spaulding EH. Chemical disinfection in the operating room. Mil Med 1958;123(6): 437–43.
15. Spaulding EH, Emmons EK. Chemical disinfection. Am J Nurs 1958;58(9): 1238–42.
16. TJC. Standards BoosterPaks™: a quality improvement tool. High-Level Disinfection (HLD) and Sterilization BoosterPak. Dec 7, 2015. Available at: https://www.jointcommission.org/standards_booster_paks/. Accessed March 7, 2019.
17. Spaulding EH. Chemical disinfection and antisepsis in the hospital. J Hosp Res 1972;9:5–31.
18. Dirlam Langlay AM, Ofstead CL, Mueller NJ, et al. Reported gastrointestinal endoscope reprocessing lapses: the tip of the iceberg. Am J Infect Control 2013;41(12):1188–94.
19. Flexible endoscopes: cleaning up the assumptions on safety 2015. Available at: https://apicintermountain.webs.com/2015%20Conference/Grace%20Thornhill_Flex%20Endo%20Oct%20%202015.pdf. Accessed March 7, 2019.
20. Alvarado CJ, Anderson AG, Maki DG. Microbiologic assessment of disposable sterile endoscopic sheaths to replace high-level disinfection in reprocessing: a prospective clinical trial with nasopharygoscopes. Am J Infect Control 2009;37(5):408–13.
21. Elackattu A, Zoccoli M, Spiegel JH, et al. A comparison of two methods for preventing cross-contamination when using flexible fiberoptic endoscopes in an otolaryngology clinic: disposable sterile sheaths versus immersion in germicidal liquid. Laryngoscope 2010;120(12):2410–6.
22. Jorgensen PH, Slotsbjerg T, Westh H, et al. A microbiological evaluation of level of disinfection for flexible cystoscopes protected by disposable endosheaths. BMC Urol 2013;13:46.
23. The Joint Commission. Reuse of single-use devices: understanding risks and strategies for decision-making for health care organizations. Oak Brook (IL): Joint Commission International; 2017.
24. Antibiotic resistance threats in the United States, 2013. Available at: www.cdc.gov/drugresistance/threat-report-2013/. Accessed March 7, 2019.
25. FDA. Infections associated with reprocessed duodenoscopes 2017. Available at: https://www.fda.gov/medicaldevices/productsandmedicalprocedures/reprocessingofreusablemedicaldevices/ucm454630.htm. Accessed July 31 2018.
26. TJC. A Joint Commission/FDA Webinar on Reprocessing of Scopes. 2015. https://www.jointcommission.org/assets/1/6/A_Joint_Commission-FDA_Webinar.pdf. Accessed March 7, 2019.
27. Ethylene oxide emissions standards for sterilization facilities: national emission standards for hazardous air pollutants (NESHAP). In: United States Environmental Protection Agency, editorvol. 40 2006. CFR Part 63 Subpart O. Available at: https://www.epa.gov/stationary-sources-air-pollution/ethylene-oxide-emissions-standards-sterilization-facilities. Accessed March 7, 2019.

28. AAMI. Citing infection danger, experts call for endoscope sterilization. Arlington (VA): American Association for Medical Instrumentation; 2017.

29. Komanduri S, Abu Dayyeh BK, Bhat YM, et al. Technologies for monitoring the quality of endoscope reprocessing. Gastrointest Endosc 2014;80(3):369–73.

30. Withdrawl of disinfectant hit by safety fears. 2018. Available at: http://news.bbc. co.uk/2/hi/health/1775534.stm. Accessed August 31, 2018.

31. AUA/SUNA. White paper on reprocessing of flexible cystoscopes 2013. Available at: http://www.auanet.org/guidelines/flexible-cystoscopes. Accessed July 30, 2018.

32. Revital-Ox™ RESERT® high level disinfectant. Available at: https://www.steris. com/healthcare/products/endoscope-reprocessing/high-level-disinfection/revital-ox-resert-high-level-disinfectant/. Accessed August 28, 2018.

33. Shellnutt C. Advances in endoscope reprocessing technology and its impact on pathogen transmission. Gastroenterol Nurs 2016;39(6):457–65.

34. OSHA. Occupational safety and health standards. Personal protective equipment. Vol 1910.132. Available at: https://www.osha.gov/laws-regs/regulations/standardnumber/1910/1910.132. Accessed March 7, 2019.

35. Ofstead CL, Horton RA, Snyder AK, et al. Factors that contribute to nonadherence with endoscope reprocessing guidelines: a prospective study 2009.

36. Alfa MJ, Nemes R, Olson N, et al. Manual methods are suboptimal compared with automated methods for cleaning of single-use biopsy forceps. Infect Control Hosp Epidemiol 2006;27(8):841–6.

37. Ofstead CL, Wetzler HP, Amelang MR, et al. Reprocessing effectiveness for gastroscopes and colonscoeps: longitudinal comparison of two methods. Presented at Society of Gastroenterology Nurses and Associates (SGNA) meeting, Seattle, Washington, May 22–24, 2016.

38. Rutala WA, Weber DJ. Guideline for disinfection and sterilization in healthcare facilities, 2008. Available at: https://www.cdc.gov/infectioncontrol/pdf/guidelines/disinfection-guidelines.pdf. Accessed March 7, 2019.

39. Kovaleva J. Endoscope drying and its pitfalls. J Hosp Infect 2017;97(4):319–28.

40. Alfa MJ, Olson N, DeGagne P. Automated washing with the Reliance Endoscope Processing System and its equivalence to optimal manual cleaning. Am J Infect Control 2006;34(9):561–70.

41. Cowen AE. The clinical risks of infection associated with endoscopy. Can J Gastroenterol 2001;15(5):321–31.

Coding for Otolaryngology Office Procedures

Richard W. Waguespack, MD[a],*, Lawrence M. Simon, MD[b]

KEYWORDS

- Coding • Correct coding • Office procedures

KEY POINTS

- Physicians must know how to correctly code for their procedures and services. Although many institutions use professional coders, physicians remain ultimately responsible for code submitted under their names.
- Codes may change on an annual basis. It is critical that every surgeon devote continuing educational time each year to keeping up with coding, including access to the most recent Current Procedural Terminology (CPT) codebook and related resources. Familiarization with introductory language often found at the beginning of each section as well as linked parentheticals, in addition to code numbers and descriptions, is highly encouraged.
- Physicians must be familiar with facility versus nonfacility reimbursement valuation as determined by the Centers for Medicare & Medicaid Services and commercial insurers and with all applicable state and federal regulations for in-office procedures.

OVERVIEW OF CURRENT PROCEDURAL TERMINOLOGY PROCESS

CPT stands for Current Procedural Terminology and is owned by the American Medical Association (AMA). The CPT code set is maintained by the CPT Editorial Panel of the AMA. The Panel is composed of 17 members: 11 physician members nominated from national medical specialty societies and chosen by the AMA Board of Trustees (with no

Disclosure Statement: The coding instructions provided herein are the opinions of the authors and are derived from the authors' experiences as members of the CPT Advisory Committee, the CPT Editorial Panel, and the *CPT Assistant* Editorial Board. They in no way represent the official opinions or views of the American Academy of Otolaryngology–Head and Neck Surgery (AAO/HNS) or any other medical society nor do they represent the opinions or views of the authors' employers. It remains the responsibility of each surgeon to accurately code their work and be familiar with all relevant payer policy.

[a] Department of Otolaryngology–Head and Neck Surgery, University of Alabama at Birmingham, 1808 7th Avenue South, BDB 563, Birmingham, AL 35233, USA; [b] LSU Health Sciences Center, Department of Otolaryngology–Head and Neck Surgery, University Hospital and Clinics, 2390 West Congress Street, Lafayette, LA 70506, USA
* Corresponding author.
E-mail address: rwaguespack@uabmc.edu

specialty-designated positions); 1 physician representative each from the Blue Cross and Blue Shield Association (BCBSA), the Centers for Medicare & Medicaid Services (CMS), the American Hospital Association (AHA), and America's Health Insurance Plans (AHIP); and 2 nonphysician representatives (eg, audiologist and occupational therapist) from the Healthcare Professionals Advisory Committee (HCPAC). The Panel is supported by the CPT Advisory Committee, which is comprised of representatives from national medical specialty societies that have a seat at the AMA House of Delegates. Each society is allotted 1 advisor and 1 advisor alternate, and these members aid the Panel by providing specialty specific input on all coding matters and education to their societal membership; they serve as liaisons between the Panel and their specialty society. Lastly, the AMA also publishes the *CPT Assistant*, which provides guidance on the interpretation and appropriate use of codes and helps answer common and/or complex coding questions. *CPT Assistant* articles[2] are edited and approved by the *CPT Assistant* Editorial Board, which has representation from the CPT Advisory Committee, the CPT Editorial Panel, the Resource Based Relative Value Scale Update Committee (RUC), CMS, BCBSA, AHIP, HCPAC, and AHA.

New codes are proposed by completing a code change application, which can be found on the AMA Web site (https://www.ama-assn.org/practice-management/CPT-current-procedural-terminology). The most common pathway for physicians to propose a new code, or modify an existing code, is to bring the matter to the relevant clinical and socioeconomic committees in their specialty societies, which then vet the idea. If the procedure is deemed to meet the criteria for a dedicated CPT code, an application is submitted to the AMA. The Panel meets 3 times a year, where it reviews applications and addresses other pending CPT matters. Other interested parties, such drug or equipment manufacturers, may submit code change applications.

MODIFIERS

The correct use of modifiers is critical to correctly reporting many procedures performed by otolaryngologists. They communicate important information about the procedure, such as whether or not it is distinct from the office evaluation and management (E/M) work and whether or not a procedure is unilateral or bilateral. The most pertinent modifiers for in-office otolaryngology procedures are as follows:

Modifier	Intended Use	Notes
25	Append to an E/M code when 1 is performed and reported on the same day as a minor procedure (defined as a procedure with a 0-d or 10-d global period) when the decision to perform the procedure (constituting an E/M visit) is on the same day as the procedure. The decision must not have been made to perform the procedure at a previous day's visit.	All procedures (even minor ones) already include some E/M work. It is not appropriate to report an E/M and use modifier −25 when all of the E/M work was related to the procedure. An example: if seeing a patient with a complaint of hearing loss, but the patient also notes nasal congestion and and it is decided that a nasal endoscopy is indicated, then appending modifier −25 to the E/M code is appropriate. If a patient comes in for known nasal obstruction or nasal débridement for which performing an endoscopy is already planned, then it is not appropriate to report an E/M with modifier −25.

(continued on next page)

(continued)		
Modifier	**Intended Use**	**Notes**
52	Reduced services modifier	Sometimes, it is medically necessary to perform only a portion of a procedure. One example is performing a bilateral procedure (eg, tonsillectomy) on only 1 side. When this happens, the surgeon should append modifier −52 to the procedure.
50	This modifier is appended to a unilateral procedure when bilateral performance is performed.	Diagnostic nasal endoscopy is already a bilateral procedure, so modifier −50 is not used with this code under any circumstance. Other surgical nasal endoscopy codes, however, are unilateral. If a patient needs to have a nasal endoscopic procedure performed on both sides, then using modifier −50 is appropriate.
57	Append this modifier to an E/M code when 1 is performed and reported on the same day as a major procedure (defined as a procedure with a 90-d global period) when the decision to perform the procedure (constituting an E/M visit) was on the same day as the procedure. The decision must not have been made to perform the procedure at a previous day's visit.	Do not use modifier −57 to bill for the E/M work of a preoperative history and physical (typically done or attested in the day of surgery). Also, remember that all procedures (even minor ones) already include some E/M work. It is not appropriate to report an E/M and use modifier −57 when all of the E/M work was related to the procedure. An example: if seeing a patient with a complaint of throat pain and the patient is found to have a peritonsillar abscess that must be drained that day (10-d global), then appending modifier −25 to the E/M code is appropriate; if a quinsy tonsillectomy were performed the same day (90-d global), the modifier is −57. If a patient comes in for a scheduled tonsillectomy, and a preoperative history and physical is simply performed on the day of surgery, then it is not appropriate to report an E/M and modifier −57.
79	This modifier is used when a procedure must be performed inside the global period of another unrelated procedure.	One common use of modifier −79 in otolaryngology is for postoperative nasal sinus débridements. If a patient has septoplasty and functional endoscopic sinus surgery (FESS), then the 90-d global period of the septoplasty overrides the 0-d global period of the FESS. If the patient needs to undergo nasal sinus endoscopy with débridement of the ethmoid cavity (ie, débridement unrelated to the septoplasty), then append modifier −79 to the nasal endoscopy with débridement code (31237), with modifier 50 if performed bilaterally, to communicate to the payer that the debridement was related to the 0-d global period FESS and not to the 90-d global period septoplasty.

OFFICE-BASED COSMETIC PROCEDURES

Most cosmetic procedures are cash-based transactions that are not billed to insurance companies, and as such, CPT codes may or may not be used. It is important to negotiate fees with patients beforehand and to be as transparent as possible about all costs. It is especially critical to disclose any hidden fees, such as anesthesia, radiology, pathology, and facility charges. This discussion becomes even more germane if part of the procedure is cosmetic and part of it functional (as may be common with combined functional and cosmetic nasal surgeries.) If part of the procedure is billed to insurance, consider network status with anticipated out-of-pocket patient cost as well and obtaining an Advanced Beneficiary Notice (ABN). An ABN is a document signed by both the physician and the patient that acknowledges that the patient accepts financial responsibility in the event that insurance does not cover the physician's fees. An example of an ABN that can be used for Medicare patients can be found at https://www.cms.gov/Medicare/Medicare-General-Information/BNI/ABN.html.

PERTINENT CLASSIFICATIONS OF OFFICE-BASED PROCEDURES WITH THEIR ATTENDANT CODES
Skin Care, Liposuction, and Hair Restoration

Procedure	Code(s)	Notes
Botulinum toxin injections	64612–64616	Can be used for botulinum toxin injections depending on which muscles are denervated. 64653 can be used if botulinum toxin is used to treat facial or cervical hyperhidrosis.
Filler injections	11950–11954	Can be used to report subcutaneous filler injection. Code selection is based on volume of filler injected. Additionally, supply code G0429 can be used to report dermal filler injection specifically to treat facial lipodystrophy syndrome (such as occurs in patients with HIV on antiretroviral therapy).
Chemical peels	15788 and 15789	Epidermal and dermal facial peels, respectively
	15792 and 15793	Nonfacial epidermal and dermal peels, respectively
	17360	Chemical peel is used specifically to treat acne
Dermabrasion	15780	Total face
	15781	Segmental, face
	15782	Regional, other than face (eg, neck)
	15783	Superficial dermabrasion, any site
Laser resurfacing	No applicable codes	No applicable CPT codes exist for cosmetic resurfacing. Codes 17106–17111 may be applicable if the laser is used to destroy either vascular or other benign lesions
Rhinophyma treatment	30120	Rhinophyma resection or resurfacing (regardless of technique)
Liposuction	15876–15879	15876 is the code for liposuction in the head and neck (such as submental). If liposuction of the trunk or extremities also is performed, use codes 15877–15879.
Hair restoration	15220–15221 15775–15776	15220 and/or 15221 is for full-thickness scalp strip transplant. If plugs/punch grafts are used, then codes 15775 and 15776 can be used, depending on how many punch grafts are placed.

Facelift

Facelift codes	15819	Specific for cervicoplasty (eg, repair of platysmal banding)
	15824–15828	The traditional facelift codes, and code selection is based on location of rhytids.
	15829	Specific for superficial musculoaponeurotic system (SMAS) flap

Rhinoplasty and Septoplasty

Rhinoplasty/ septorhinoplasty	30400–30462	Cosmetic or functional rhinoplasty/septorhinoplasty, depending on what work is performed
Internal nasal valve repair	30465	This code can be reported with the rhinoplasty codes if a spreader graft or alar batten graft is placed in addition to the rhinoplasty. Also, this is a bilateral code. If only 1 nostril is addressed, then append the reduced services modifier (modifier −52) to the code.
Septoplasty	30520	Can be reported with all rhinoplasty codes except for 30420, which includes major septal repair. If a septorhinoplasty is performed, use 30420 and do not separately report the septoplasty with 30520.
Unlisted procedure, nose	30999	Use this code to report treatment nasal valve collapse with various techniques designed to create scarring and rigidity in the lateral wall (eg, *radiofrequency lesions and/or absorbable polymer implants*).

- Coding tip: 20912 is used to report harvest of septal cartilage graft (such as for ear reconstruction). If a septoplasty also is performed and reported, the the septal graft harvest should not be separately reported.
- Coding tip: the codes for open treatment of nasal bone and/or nasal septal fractures (21325, 21330, 21335, and 21336) cannot be used to report rhinoplasty. These codes are only appropriate for the treatment of acute fractures. Treatment of healed fractures with osteotomies and further modification is reported with the rhinoplasty code set, even if the deformity being treated is the result of a prior fracture.

CODES FOR BLEPHAROPLASTY, BROW LIFT, AND OTHER OCULAR PROCEDURES (INCLUDING GOLD WEIGHT PLACEMENT)

Cosmetic Blepharoplasty	15820–15823	Cosmetic blepharoplasty. Codes 15820 and 15821 are used for lower eyelid. 15822 and 15823 are used for upper eyelid.
Direct brow lift	67900	Brow lift performed to correct brow ptosis (as opposed to forehead rhytidectomy, which is reported with 15824).
Functional treatment of ptosis	67901–67908	Repair of blepharoptosis. Code selection is based on technique.
	67909	Reduction of overcorrection of ptosis
Lid retraction	67911	Correction of lid retraction
Lagophthalmos	67912	Correction of lagophthalmos with implantation of an upper lid load. This code is used for gold weight placement in a patient with facial nerve palsy.

MOHS RECONSTRUCTION AND SCAR REVISION (LESION CODES)

Excision is reported by the Mohs surgeon separately.

Intermediate and Complex Repair Codes

Intermediate and complex repair codes are used when a wound is reconstructed using undermining and layered closure. When using these codes, refer to the latest edition of

CPT Professional Edition[1] for instruction on how to differentiate intermediate versus complex wound closures. Layered closure usually is considered an intermediate closure. Extensive undermining, scar revision, débridement, and the need for stents and/or retention sutures are the criteria for complex closure.

The coding of repairs is differentiated further by location and size of the defect (not the size of the lesion that was excised.) When multiple defects from the same anatomic area and level of complexity are repaired, do not report them separately. Instead, add up their lengths and use the sum to select the correct codes.

Lastly, the complex repair codes have 2 key differences from the intermediate range. First, full-thickness repairs of the lips and eyelids are not included in the complex repair section. Second, defects larger than 7.5 cm are reported using an add-on code for each additional 5 cm (or less) over 7.5 cm.

Procedure	Code(s)	Notes
Intermediate repair codes—select based on size and location	12031–12037	Scalp
	12041–12047	Neck
	12051–12057	Face, ears, eyelids, nose, lips, and/or mucous membranes
Complex repair codes—select based on size and location	13120–13122	Scalp
	13131–13133	Forehead, cheeks, chin, mouth, and/or neck
	13151–13153	Eyelids, nose, ears, and/or lips

- Full-thickness repairs of the lips are reported with 40650 to 40654.
- Eyelid repairs that involve the lid margin, tarsus, and/or palpebral conjunctiva are reported with 67930.
- Full-thickness eyelid repairs are reported with 67935.

Adjacent Tissue Transfers (Local Flaps Without a Vascular Pedicle [eg, Bilobe and Rhomboid Flaps])

CPT codes 14000 to 14302 include the work of the lesion resection if performed by the same surgeon. If the resecting surgeon and the reconstructing surgeon perform both portions together, then both surgeons should only report the tissue transfer code with modifier −62 (the cosurgeon modifier). If 1 surgeon does the resection and 1 surgeon performs the reconstruction, then each uses separate codes to report that surgeon's portion of the procedure. Some key points to remember:

- As with the complex repair codes, full-thickness repairs of eyelids and lips are reported with their respective codes (outlined previously).
- The key maneuver that differentiates adjacent tissue transfers (the CPT term for local flaps) from complex closure is that additional incisions are made; refer to the introductory language in the Adjacent Tissue Transfer or Rearrangement section of the Integumentary System.[1]
- If a skin graft is necessary to close the donor site, it is reported separately.
- Repair codes are chosen based on the location and size of the defect. The location-specific codes are divided into codes for 10 cm^2 or less and 10.1 cm^2 to 30 cm^2. There are non–site-specific codes for 30.1 cm^2 to 60 cm^2 and an add-on code used for each additional 30 cm^2.
- The defect size is determined by adding the sizes of both the primary defect of the excision and the secondary defect that the flap design creates.

Adjacent Tissue Transfer Codes

Procedure	Code(s)	Notes
Local flap procedures (based on location)	14020 and 14021	Scalp reconstruction
	14040 and 14041	Reconstruction of forehead, cheeks, chin, mouth, and/or neck
	14060 and 14061	Reconstruction of eyelid, nose, ears, and/or lips
	14301	Reconstruction of any area, 30.1–60 cm^2
	+14302	Any area, each addition 30 cm^2 or part thereof
These codes are to report local flaps without a major vascular pedicle (eg, bilobe and rhomboid flaps)		

- Coding tip: a code with the + sign is an add-on and must be used with another primary code. Look for parenthetic information to determine circumstances under which the add-on can or cannot be used.

Pedicled Flaps and Composite Grafts

Pedicled flaps and composite grafts procedures are differentiated by site of defect, site of flap harvest, composition of the flap, and whether or not there is a named major vascular pedicle. A full discussion of all of these codes is beyond the scope of this article, but those pertinent to office work are discussed herein. Lastly, donor site repair by skin graft or local flap (adjacent tissue transfer) is reported separately. The pertinent codes to consider are as follows:

Procedure	Code(s)	Notes
Pedicled delayed inset flaps	15572–15576	Formation of a direct or tubed pedicle (used when the flap is formed but not transferred into the donor site at the time of reporting)—scalp (15572); forehead, cheeks, chin, mouth, and/or neck (15574); and eyelids, nose, ears, lips, intraoral (15576)
	15620 and 15630	Delay of a flap or sectioning of a flap with division and inset at forehead, cheeks, chin, and/or neck (15620); and eyelids, nose, ears, and/or lips (15630). Report based on donor site of flap (location of division/sectioning of flap)
Specific pedicled head and neck flaps	15730	Midface flap (this is the traditional midface or cervical advancement flap, also called the zygomaticofacial flap). This flap does not have a single, named, major vascular pedicle, but it involves the preservation of the blood supply at the base of the flap.
	15731	Paramedian forehead flap
	15733	Other head and neck local flaps that have recognized, named, major vascular pedicles. The code provides an exclusive list of the flaps that are included in this code. They are buccinator, genioglossus, temporalis, masseter, sternocleidomastoid, and levator scapulae.
Island pedicle flaps	15740 and 15750	Island pedicle flaps. 15740 requires the dissection and preservation of an anatomically named major axial vessel. 15750 is used when the pedicle is neurovascular.
Composite grafts	15760	Composite (full-thickness) graft. Examples include a full-thickness graft from the external ear or nasal ala.
	15770	Composite dermal-fat-fascia graft

- Coding tip: +15777, the add-on code for biologic implant placement, is now restricted to use in the breast and trunk. For placement of a biologic implant in the head and neck, use 17999.

Skin Grafts and Skin Replacement Surgery

In performing skin grafts and skin replacement surgery procedures, there are separate codes for wound (recipient site) preparation and for the graft replacement. The codes for wound preparation, however, are unlikely to be used if reconstruction is done in the same setting as the Mohs resection. The wound bed already is ready. In terms of the graft, the correct code is chosen based on type of skin graft used and the location and size of the recipient wound (not of the skin graft harvested). There also are separate codes for the application of nonautologous tissue and skin substitute grafts (eg, cadaveric skin), but do not use these codes to report for application of nongraft wound dressings (eg, petroleum gauze and a dry gauze wrap). Other key points are

- For grafting of multiple wounds from the same anatomic site grouping, use the sum of the wound defect sizes to select the proper code.
- Full-thickness skin graft codes include direct closure of the donor site.

Skin Grafts and Skin Replacement Surgery

Procedure	Code(s)	Notes
Wound preparation	15004 and +15005	Wound preparation. Not likely to be used unless the skin graft is used as a delayed closure (ie, at a different operative setting from the Mohs resection)
Various skin grafting codes. Code selection depends on type, size, and location of skin graft performed.	15115 and +15116	Epidermal autograft to face, scalp, eyelids, mouth, neck, ears, and/or orbits. 15115 is for the first 100 cm^2 in patients 10 y of age and older or the first 1% of body surface area (BSA) in patients younger than 10 y of age. 15116 is for each additional 100 cm^2 or 1% BSA or part thereof.
	15120 and +15121	Split-thickness autograft to face, scalp, eyelids, mouth, neck, ears, and/or orbits. 15120 is for the first cm^2 in patients 10 y of age and older or the first 1% of BSA in patients younger than 10 y of age. 15121 is for each additional 100 cm^2 or 1% of BSA or part thereof.
	15135 and +15136	Dermal autograft to face, scalp, eyelids, mouth, neck, ears, and/or orbits. 15135 is for the first 100 cm^2 in patients 10 y of age and older or the first 1% of BSA in patients younger than 10 y of age. 15136 is for each additional 100 cm^2 or 1% of BSA or part thereof.
	15220 and +15221	Full-thickness skin graft, scalp. 15220 is for 20 cm^2 or less. +15221 is for each additional 20 cm^2 or part thereof.
	15240 and +15241	Full-thickness skin graft, forehead, cheeks, chin, mouth, and/or neck. 15240 is for 20 cm^2 or less. +15241 is for each additional 20 cm^2 or part thereof.
	15260 and 15261	Full-thickness skin graft, nose, ears, eyelids, and/or lips. 15260 is for 20 cm^2 or less. +15261 is for each additional 20 cm^2 or part thereof.

(continued on next page)

Procedure	Code(s)	Notes
(continued)		
Skin substitute (nonautogenous) graft placement	15275, +15276, 15277 and + 15278	Application of skin substitute graft to face, scalp, eyelids, mouth, neck, ears, and/or orbits. 15275 and +15276 are for wounds up to 100 total cm^2. 15275 is for the first 25 cm^2, and +15276 is for each additional 25 cm^2 or part thereof. For wounds equal to or larger than 100 cm^2, use codes 15277 and +15278. 15277 is for the first 100 cm^2, and +15278 is for each additional 100 cm^2 or part thereof.
Other miscellaneous graft codes	20900	Harvesting of bone graft, any donor area, minor/small
	20910	Harvesting of costochondral graft
	20912	Harvest of septal cartilage graft (may not be reported with septoplasty)
	20926	Tissue grafts, other (eg, partenon, fat, or dermis.) This code could be used for harvesting abdominal fat, ear lobe fat, or temporalis fascia, as examples.

OFFICE-BASED SINUS PROCEDURES

Office sinus procedures are reported using the same codes as in the operating room. Reimbursement may vary, however, depending on whether or not an office or clinic is considered a facility. This distinction may be important for doctors who work in academic centers and/or hospital-owned outpatient facilities.

In sinus surgical coding, the guiding principle is that only 1 code can be billed for any 1 sinus in a single surgical session, and the most extensive code is the 1 that is reported. For example, irrigation of the right maxillary sinus cannot be billed with balloon dilation of the maxillary sinus or maxillary antrostomy of this sinus. Only the primary and definitive dilation or antrostomy should be reported.

Office-Based Nasal and Sinus Procedures

Procedure	Code(s)	Notes
Nasal foreign body	30300	Removal of nasal foreign body, without general anesthesia. This code is independent of the type of instrument used. This code is used for both unilateral and bilateral nasal foreign bodies. Modifier −50 may not be used for bilateral work, but modifier −52 does not need to be appended if only a unilateral foreign body is removed.
Diagnostic nasal endoscopy	31231	Diagnostic nasal endoscopy. Note that the introductory language to nasal endoscopy states that the procedure includes inspection of the interior of the nasal cavity and the middle and superior meatus, the turbinates, and the sphenoethmoid recess. If it is not possible to access and visualize all of these areas, then a reduced services modifier (modifier −52) must be appended to the code.

(continued on next page)

(continued)

Procedure	Code(s)	Notes
Destruction of an intranasal lesion	30117	This code currently is used by many otolaryngologists to report nasal swell body destruction. It is important to remember that this is a classically open code. Although the code is valued as an endoscopic code, its use for endoscopic procedures is new. As such, some coders may recommend that surgeons report swell body reduction with the unlisted nasal procedure code 30999, and this is also correct. 30117 should not be reported separately to treat swell bodies if a septoplasty is concurrently performed.
Functional endoscopic sinus surgery and endoscopic nasal débridement/biopsy/polypectomy	31237	Nasal endoscopy with biopsy, polypectomy, or débridement Use modifier −50 if bilateral work is performed. Be sure to document medical necessity for performing a débridement Use modifier −79 if the patient also underwent a septoplasty within the prior 90 d Do not report with any functional endoscopic sinus surgery code on the same side of the nose (31240–31288 [excluding 31241]) during the same operative session
	31240–31288 (excluding 31241)	Endoscopic sinus surgery codes. These are increasingly performed in the office. Use modifier −50 if performed bilaterally. Coding tip: CPT codes 31259, 31267, and 31288 are used to report the work of removing significant amounts of tissue from within the sinus. Removing the tissue of the lateral nasal wall and some polypoid mucosa from within the maxillary sinus is insufficient to report 31267. The same axiom holds true for 31259 and 31288 with regard to the sphenoid sinus. The phrase, "with removal of tissue," in 31259, 31267, and 31288 connotes that a significant amount of material (such as a tumor, polyp, or allergic fungal mucin) was removed from the inside of the sinus, not just at the peristomal region. Refer to instructions in *CPT Assistant*[2] and the CPT for ENT published by the American Academy of Otolaryngology–Head and Neck Surgery for more information on the correct use of these codes.
Sinus ostial dilation	31295–31298	These codes are used to report sinus ostial dilation of the maxillary, sphenoid, or frontal sinuses or a combination of the frontal and sphenoid sinuses. Dilation is typically, but not exclusively, performed using a balloon.

(continued on next page)

(continued)

Procedure	Code(s)	Notes
Inferior turbinate surgery	30140 and 30802	These are the codes used to report either submucous resection (30140) or ablation (30802) of the inferior turbinates. 30140 is a unilateral code. If both turbinates are resected, then append modifier −50. 30802 is an inherently bilateral code. If only 1 turbinate is ablated, then use modifier −52. Do not separately report turbinate out- (or lateral) fracture (30930) or nasal endoscopy (31231) with either code. Note that both codes are submucosal. If mucosa is resected or ablated, use 30130 or 30801, respectively. Typical uses of 30140 include the microdébrider or sickle knife and sinus instruments. Typical uses of 30802 include radiofrequency ablation and similar methodologies. Coding tip: suction removal of ablated tissue is considered resection for purposes of using 30140. Use of a device that ablates tissue and only evacuates blood or plume is still reported with 30802.
Unlisted procedure, accessory sinuses	31299	Unlisted procedure, accessory sinuses. This code can have many uses. If it is used for a procedure, be sure to also submit a comparison code that represents similar work and can be used as a benchmark for payment. More instructions on the use of unlisted codes can be found on the American Academy of Otolaryngology–Head and Neck Surgery Web site. One common example of the use of this unlisted code, at the time of this publication, is the placement of a drug-eluting nasal/sinus stent or implant into the maxillary, ethmoid, frontal, or sphenoid sinuses at a different session from a primary surgery (eg, 31237, 31240, 31253–31288). When using drug-eluting implants, S1090 and J3490 also sometimes are used to report the devices themselves. Check with local payers to see what their specific policies are regarding these devices.

Epistaxis

Procedure	Code(s)	Notes
Non-endoscopic control of epistaxis	30901-30906	These codes are used for management of epistaxis without nasal endoscopy. CPT code 30901 would be used for simple control of anterior bleeding (such as silver nitrate cautery of the anterior septum and packing). CPT code 30903 would be used for more complex control of anterior bleeding, which extensive cautery and/or packing is needed. Codes 30901 and 30902 are unilateral codes and may be reported with modifier 50.

(continued on next page)

Procedure	Code(s)	Notes
(continued)		
		CPT code 30905 would be used for the initial control of posterior nasal bleeding with posterior packing and/or cautery of any kind, and CPT code 30906 would be used if the same episode of epistaxis requires subsequent packing. Posterior packing is typically placed into the very posterior nasal cavity and/or into the nasopharynx. These codes are generally not reported bilaterally with modifier 50. Of note, these codes should not be reported for control of bleeding during nasal or sinus surgery; control of intraoperative bleeding is inherent to the primary surgery.
Endoscopic control of epistaxis	31238	This code would be used to report endoscopic control of either anterior or posterior bleeding with any method, such as cautery and/or packing. An example would be the use of suction cautery or silver nitrate performed using endoscopic guidance, typically with a rigid nasal endoscope. As noted above, this code should not be reported for control of bleeding during nasal or sinus surgery.
Endoscopic ligation of the sphenopalatine artery	31241	This code describes endoscopic sphenopalatine artery ligation, which is uncommonly performed in the office. It is intended to treat primary epistaxis and requires endoscopic dissection and exposure of the sphenopalatine artery with ligation of this artery. It should not be reported for control of bleeding associated with primary endoscopic sinus surgery or any control of bleeding that does not involve identification and ligation of the sphenopalatine artery.

IN-OFFICE FUNCTIONAL NASAL SURGERY

Many of the in-office functional nasal surgery procedures are discussed previously. Inferior turbinate resection and reduction procedures are discussed previously. Additionally, standard septoplasty and rhinoplasty procedures are reporting using the same codes as used in the operating room (30400–30462 and 30520). Lastly, there are myriad nasal valve procedures, some of which are reported with 30465, and many others are reported using 30999.

- 30465: this code is used to report surgical repair of nasal vestibular stenosis. It is a bilateral code (like tonsillectomy), and modifier −52 should be used when only 1 nostril is addressed. As currently valued, this code should be used only when some sort of cartilaginous graft (such as a spreader or batten graft) is placed or some sort of significant work (such as suturing and/or excision) is performed on the nasal cartilage. It is not appropriate to use this code for shorter in-office techniques, with or without an implant, to strengthen the nasal side wall and prevent valve collapse.
- 30999: this is the appropriate code to use for the various procedures currently used to treat nasal valve stenosis through strengthening the nasal sidewall. Examples may include the placement of an absorbable nasal implant and/or the creation of radiofrequency or electrocautery lesions in the nasal side wall or nasal ala.

OFFICE-BASED OTOLOGY PROCEDURES

A considerable amount of otology is performed in the office setting. There are a few essential codes and concepts to know and understand about these procedures.

Otoendoscopy (Diagnostic)

Routine otoscopy is included in the E/M work of a patient visit. If extensive diagnostic otoendoscopy is performed, however, it is reported with the appropriate unlisted ear code (69399 for external ear if only the canal is visualized and 69799 if the middle ear is visualized). Bear in mind that the clinic note needs to substantiate the medical necessity of an ear examination that is more extensive than standard otoscopy and otomicroscopy, and a separate procedure note needs to be generated. Also, if a procedure is performed, the endoscopy is bundled with the procedure and not separately reported.

Key In-office Otology Codes

Procedure	Code(s)	Notes
Hematoma/abscess drainage	-69005	Drainage of auricular hematoma or abscess. 69000 is simple drainage and includes dressing, when used (eg, aspiration, simple incision, application of straightforward dressing). 69005 is complex drainage (eg, extended incision with dissection of loculations, placement of a complex sutured bolster dressing). Both have 10-d globals.
Ear tube–related procedures	69420	Myringotomy without tube placement. Can be performed with topical/local and includes aspiration and/or irrigation, if performed. This code is unilateral and modifier −50 can be used if the procedure is performed bilaterally.
	69424	This is the code for ear tube removal. This code is never be used in the office, because it requires the use of general anesthesia. Removal of a tympanostomy tube with replacement is reported with the appropriate tube placement code; If only the tube is removed without general anesthesia, the appropriate level E/M code is reported.
	69433	This code is for placement of pressure equalizing ear (tympanostomy) tubes that does not require general anesthesia. This code is not site-specific or service-specific, only that general anesthesia is not utilized. As such, it is most likely the code that is used for placement of ear tubes in the office. This code includes use of the operating microscope and is a unilateral code. If the procedure is performed in both ears, the modifier −50 can be used. And do not separately report removal of impacted cerumen 69210.
Ear foreign body removal	69200	Foreign body removal from the external auditory canal without general anesthesia. If cerumen is removed with the foreign body, it is bundled with the foreign body removal. The code is unilateral, so modifier −50 can be used if foreign bodies are removed from both ears. *Ear tubes are not considered foreign bodies in this context.*

(continued on next page)

(continued)

Procedure	Code(s)	Notes
Cerumen removal	69210	Removal of impacted cerumen. The key to the use of this code is to document both the removal of impacted cerumen with instrumentation and the medical necessity of removing the cerumen. Further information on the correct use of this code can be found in *CPT Assistant*[2] and on the CPT for ENT site of the American Academy of Otolaryngology–Head and Neck Surgery (https://www.entnet.org/content/CPT®-ent-cerumen-removal)
Myringoplasty (tympanic membrane repair without elevation of a tympano meatal flap)	69610	Use this code when a tissue graft is not harvested. This code is appropriate for the use of a paper or hyaluronic acid disk patch.
	69620	Use this code is when a donor site is used for a graft, such as fat or tragal cartilage. Two classic examples of this code are a fat-graft and a cartilage butterfly graft. This code is not used if a tympanomeatal flap is elevated. *The graft harvest is not reported separately.*
Labyrinthotomy with perfusion (transtympanic injection)	69801	This code may be used to report transtympanic membrane injections of cochleoactive and vestibuloactive substances. Examples include transtympanic injections of steroids and gentamycin. The medication is reported separately. If an ear tube is placed at the same time as the injection, only the injection is reported.
Mastoid bowl cleaning/ débridement	69220 and 69222	Mastoid débridement, simple and complex. The CPT descriptors are somewhat nebulous about the distinction between simple and complex, although the latter is supported if anesthesia is used. Be sure that documentation supports the procedure, complexity, and its medical necessity. Medical necessity for work independent of the mastoid débridement must be demonstrated if this code is used with an E/M service. If the documentation supports a separate E/M (for example, for prescription management of a nonotologic complaint), then it is appropriate to use modifier −25 with the E/M.
Binocular microscopy	92504	This code is specific for diagnostic binocular microscopy. Although payer policy may vary in regards to this code, it is correct coding to report it with 69210 when the microscope is used to remove the cerumen impaction.

The codes for myringoplasty deserve special attention. The pertinent codes are 69610 and 69620, and they represent 2 different techniques of myringoplasty, which is repair of a tympanic membrane perforation without elevation of a tympanomeatal flap. This procedure can take many forms, including paper patch, fat graft, synthetic graft such as hyaluronic acid, and cartilage butterfly graft, to name a few. The correct use of these codes is as follows:

- 69610 is used when a tissue graft is not harvested. This code is appropriate for the use of a paper or hyaluronic acid disk patch.

- 69620 is used when a donor site is used for a graft, such as fat or tragal cartilage. Two classic examples of this code are a fat-graft and a cartilage butterfly graft. This code is not used if a tympanomeatal flap is elevated. *The graft harvest is not reported separately.*

Lastly, 2 other otology codes must be addressed. They are almost exclusively used in the operating room, but there is sometimes confusion surrounding their use in the office.

- 20926 is used if the graft that is harvested for the tympanic membrane repair must be harvested through a separate incision. 20926 should not be used to report graft harvest with 69620 because the latter code includes obtaining the graft.
- +69990: this code is for use of microsurgical technique and does not include the use of loupes and equivalent magnification. It is extremely unlikely that this code is ever used in the office. Furthermore, the work associated with use of the operating microscope is included in the work of tympanoplasties and mastoidectomies and usually not eligible for separate reporting.

IN-OFFICE EUSTACHIAN TUBOPLASTY WITH ENDOSCOPE

This type of procedure (eg, balloon dilation and injection of material to close the eustachian tube) is correctly reported only with an unlisted code. Most appropriately either 42999 (unlisted procedure, pharynx, adenoids, or tonsils) or 69799 (unlisted procedure, middle ear) should be reported; although transnasal in approach, 31299 would be a less appropriate code since this is not a primary nasal sinus procedure and relates more to the nasopharynx and middle ear. Be sure to submit a comparator code that represents similar work and can be used for valuation. 31297 (nasal/sinus endoscopy, surgical; with dilation of sphenoid sinus ostium [eg, balloon dilation]) is one of the more commonly used comparator codes for this purpose.

IN-OFFICE LARNGOLOGY INJECTABLES

There are 4 primary ways to perform a laryngeal injection: indirect laryngoscopy, flexible laryngoscopy, electromyography (EMG)-directed percutaneous, and direct laryngoscopy. The latter method is not generally performed in the office.

Indirect laryngoscopy can be performed either with a mirror or with a peroral angled (70° or 90°) rigid rod telescope. Flexible laryngoscopy can be performed with either a fiberoptic or distal chip flexible laryngoscope, with or without a video tower and/or operating channel. Typically, augmentation materials are too thick to be injected via a channeled laryngoscope but the scope may act to visualize a percutaneous injection.

The larynx contains both midline and paired unilateral structures. Which structures are midline and which are paired are delineated in the introductory language of the larynx endoscopy section of the CPT codebook.[1] When procedures are performed on both paired structures (such as both arytenoids or both vocal folds) or on lesions on both sides of the larynx, then modifier −50 can be used with 31572, 31573, and 31574.

In-Office Larngology and Other Injectables

Procedure	Code(s)	Notes
Diagnostic flexible laryngoscopy	31575	Diagnostic flexible laryngoscopy. May be performed with either a fiberoptic or distal chip flexible laryngoscope.
	31579	Laryngeal stroboscopy. May be performed with either a flexible (fiberoptic or distal chip) laryngoscope or rigid telescope (angled 70° or 90°).
Indirect laryngoscopy with injection	31513	Indirect laryngoscopy with vocal cord injection. To be used when a laryngeal injection is performed using indirect laryngoscopy for guidance. The injection can be performed either percutaneously or transorally.
Flexible laryngoscopy injection procedures	31573	Therapeutic injection performed via flexible laryngoscope. The injection can be performed either percutaneously, transorally with a curved needle or via the working channel of the flexible laryngoscope. Also, the injection is meant to be therapeutic, meaning it delivers medicine that is intended to have an effect on the structure/lesion being injected. Examples include a corticosteroid injection into a granuloma, cidofovir into a papilloma, and botulinum toxin into a dystonic laryngeal muscle. The medication injected is separately reported. If the injection is performed in a facility or hospital owned clinic, be sure to comply with all pertinent regulations.
	31574	Augmentation injection performed with a flexible laryngoscope. The injection can be performed either percutaneously or transorally with a curved needle while visualizing with the flexible laryngoscope. The injection is meant to be an augmentation (eg, bulking up and/or medializing vocal cords). If the procedure is performed in a physician's office (ie, not in a facility or hospital owned practice), the injected material is not separately reported. The nonfacility value of the code includes payment for the material being injected based on Resource Based Relative Value Scale Update Committee/CMS valuation. If the injection is performed in a facility or hospital owned clinic, be sure to comply with all pertinent regulations.
Salivary gland chemodenervation (eg, for aspiration)	64611	Chemodenervation of parotid and submandibular salivary glands, bilateral. Botulinum toxin is most frequently used and is separately reportable using a supply code. Also, if all 4 glands are not injected, then modifier 52 is used. If imaging guidance is used, it is separately reportable.
Laryngeal chemodenervation (eg, with botulinum toxin)	64617	Use this code to report percutaneous laryngeal chemodenervation (such as with botulinum toxin) when no laryngoscopy is used. This code includes EMG when performed, and is not separately reportable. Remember that Medicare and some commercial payers allow wastage of botulinum toxin to be reported. The code includes chemodenervation of all muscles on 1 side of the larynx; when performed on both sides of the larynx (1 or more muscles on each side), modifier 50 should be appended. If the injection is being performed in a facility or hospital-owned clinic, be sure to comply with all pertinent regulations.
	95865	Diagnostic needle electrode laryngeal EMG is reported with 95865 needle EMG; larynx. This code can be used for diagnostic EMG of the laryngeal muscles but cannot be reported with 64617

(continued on next page)

(continued)		
Procedure	**Code(s)**	**Notes**
Ultrasound guidance for needle placement	76942	Use this code to report the use of ultrasound for needle placement, such as into a salivary gland for chemodenervation. A separate report/interpretation must be documented. Be sure to use modifier 26 (designates billing only for the physician work and not for any equipment) if the otolaryngologist does not own the ultrasound equipment.

Some Typical Supply Codes

J0585–J0588	Various botulinum toxins
J3300–J3303	Various triamcinolone formulations
J1094–J1100	Various dexamethasone formulations
J0740	Cidofovir

This list is not all inclusive and may change over time. Always be sure to confirm correct coding before submitting any claims.

Coding tip: CPT code 31575 is never considered a part of the laryngeal examination. It is diagnostic procedure performed when the larynx cannot be properly examined through traditional physical examination techniques. Typically, a failed mirror examination should be documented, and the history must reflect the laryngeal complaints that are being investigated. Flexible laryngoscopy includes visualization of the larynx, hypopharynx, and base of tongue, and the procedure note should reflect examining each of these areas. Lastly, if a patient is seen only for the follow-up of a known, stable laryngeal complaint (such as routine laryngeal cancer surveillance when the patient has no evidence of disease and no other concerns), then the E/M work of the visit is included in the laryngoscopy, and only 31575 is reported. If other work must be performed, such as a change of treatment or addressing a nonlaryngeal complaint, then an appropriate level E/M code is reported with modifier −25.

Coding tip: do not use CPT codes 31570/31571 (direct laryngoscopy with injection with or without telescope/microscope, respectively) for laryngoscopy procedures performed in the office setting.

OFFICE-BASED MANAGEMENT OF LARYNGEAL NEOPLASMS

Laryngeal neoplasms may be addressed with biopsy, removal, or destruction in the clinic/office setting. As with the injectables, there are codes for performing these procedures with either indirect (very uncommon) or flexible laryngoscopy (fiberoptic or distal chip). Modifier −50 can be used with 31572 only. Lastly, the procedures can be performed either transorally with curved instruments or via the working channel of a flexible laryngoscope when available. Coders are to note that several of these codes are out of sequence in the CPT codebook,[1] meaning that they are not in numerical order. The # symbol is used to identify codes that are listed out of numerical sequence (see "Appendix N" in the CPT codebook[1]).

Office-Based Management of Laryngeal Neoplasms

Procedure	Code(s)	Notes
Indirect laryngoscopy procedures	31510	Indirect laryngoscopy with biopsy
	31512	Indirect laryngoscopy with removal of lesion. This code is used for a complete lesion excision.
Flexible laryngoscopy destruction/ablation with laser	31572	Flexible laryngoscopy with laser destruction of a lesion. Examples include a granuloma or papilloma. Modifier −50 can be used if lesions on both of any of the paired laryngeal structures are ablated. Destruction on the same side includes biopsy. If the procedure is performed in a physician's office (ie, not in a facility or hospital owned practice), the laser fiber is not separately billed. The nonfacility value of the code includes payment for the laser fiber. If the procedure is performed in a facility or hospital owned clinic, be sure to comply with all pertinent regulations
Nonlaser based flexible laryngoscopy procedures	31576	Flexible laryngoscopy with biopsy. Note that the text of the code states "biopy(sies)" meaning that only 1 unit of the code can be reported, regardless of the number of biopsies, and modifier −50 cannot be used.
	31578	Flexible laryngoscopy with removal of lesion(s), nonlaser. This code is used for a complete lesion excision by any method other than lasering.

ULTRASOUND OF THE THYROID AND NECK

There are 2 primary codes that are used for ultrasound procedures of the neck.

The first is 76536: this code is used to report standard diagnostic ultrasound of the head and neck. This code is used for thyroid, parathyroid, and/or salivary gland ultrasound as well as any other structure in the head and neck. The code does not specify complete or limited, and it uses "e.g." in the parenthetic instruction. These details imply that meaning that this same code is used whether all structures in the head and neck are visualized or only a select few.

- Coding tip: when billing an imaging code, an otolaryngologist is held to the same documentation requirements as a radiologist. Therefore, be sure that to dictate a full imaging report of the ultrasound that is independent of any other documentation on the patient from that date of service. Also be familiar with local payer policy and regulations regarding storage and submission of pertinent images/videos. Lastly, not all states and payers recognize the ability of otolaryngologists to bill for imaging. Therefore, prior to submitting bills for the interpretation of ultrasound, be sure to meet the credentialing requirements of both the state medical licensing board and the most common payers.
- Coding tip: Use modifier −26 (professional services only) with this code if only billing for the radiological supervision and interpretation of the ultrasound. Only bill the full code without modifier −26 if a practice purchased the equipment. Do not use the code without a modifier 26 if using equipment purchased and staffed by a facility.
- Coding tip: if billing for the interpretation of the imaging guidance and/or the diagnostic ultrasound and use modifier −26 in a facility where all images are sent to

radiology, be sure to communicate with the radiology department. If both the otolaryngologist and the radiologist bill for the interpretation of the same image, commonly only 1 physician is reimbursed. If a radiologist renders a report, the otolaryngologist may capture the work of the reading in the medical decision-making portion of the E/M service for which the imaging was integral. If the otolaryngologist renders the definitive report, the most common solution is for the facility to bill with modifier −TC (technical component) to report the technical equipment used, whereas the otolaryngologist bills modifier −26 for the interpretation.

The second pertinent ultrasound code is 79642: this code is used to report the use of ultrasound to guide needle placement for another procedure (such as injection, aspiration, or biopsy). The same coding tips, discussed previously, apply to this code as to 76536. Additionally, there is an extensive list of codes with which this code (76942) cannot be used because the text of the code reads "includes imaging guidance" or other similar language. For example, the fine-needle aspiration (FNA) code set has codes that indicate the use of imaging guidance. If ultrasound was used to localize the thyroid nodule and perform the FNA, the FNA code that included imaging guidance and not 76942 is used. Again, use of modifier −26 may apply if the provider performing the FNA did not purchase the equipment being used.

Lastly, there is some controversy regarding the reporting of 76536 and 76942 by the same surgeon on the same day. From a pure CPT standpoint, it is appropriate to bill both these codes if performing a comprehensive neck and thyroid ultrasound in addition to image guidance FNA. Documentation is needed to substantiate both the performance of and medical necessity for both imaging techniques, with particular attention paid to the imaging work that did not overlap. Payer policy regarding these codes, varies, however, and many may not allow these code pairs to be used on the same date of service.

FINE-NEEDLE ASPIRATION

The foundation for coding Fine Needle Aspiration (FNA) biopsies is that they may be performed without image guidance or with modality-specific guidance. There is a dedicated code for FNA done without any kind of imaging guidance, first lesion (10021) and another code for each additional lesion that is biopsied in this fashion (#+10004). Each lesion is only reported once, regardless of the number of sticks/passes made into the lesion. There are then similarly constructed codes for first and additional lesions biopsied via FNA using ultrasound, fluoroscopy, CT guidance, and magnetic resonance guidance. In practice, only the ultrasound codes are likely applicable to the office setting by otolaryngologists. The pertinent codes are as follows:

Procedure	Code(s)	Notes
FNA with ultrasound guidance	10005	First lesion—this code is used for ultrasound-guided FNA of a lesion. It is reported once, regardless of the number of passes that are made into the lesion.
	10006	This code is used for each addition lesion that is biopsied. Report the code once per lesion, regardless of the number of needle passes made.
Coding tip: do not use 76942 with these codes. They include the use of imaging guidance.		

IN-OFFICE EVALUATION AND MANAGEMENT OF DYSPHAGIA

There are 3 tests performed with a flexible laryngoscope: flexible endoscopic evaluation of swallowing (FEES), flexible endoscopic evaluation and laryngeal sensory testing (FEEST), and FEES and laryngeal sensory testing (FEESST). This trio of services must be performed with cine recording or video recording, and each is fully described by 2 codes—1 for the performance of the test and the second for the interpretation and report. The rationale is that the endoscopic evaluation may be performed by a qualified speech therapist/speech-language pathologist (SLP) and subsequently interpreted and reported by a physician; or the physician may do both elements. The pertinent codes are as follows:

FEES	Reported with the code pair 92612 and 92613
FEEST	Reported with the code pair 92614 and 92615
FEESST	Reported with the code pair 92616 and 92617

If the examination is not recorded, the correct reporting for these is the unlisted code 92700.

Contrast esophagram (barium swallow) and modified barium swallows rarely are done in the office. Typically, the contrast esophagram (barium swallow) is performed by a radiologist and staff in an imaging suite, and billing is partitioned between the professional component (modifier 26) provided by the radiologist and the technical component representing the staff and equipment used for the study. If the interpreting doctor owns the equipment and employs the staff, the entire code is reported without modifier.

With modified barium swallows, a speech therapist or SLP is present working with the radiologist and administering different consistencies of ingestants, often with use of maneuvers to demonstrate dysphagia and potential improvements in swallowing (chin tuck, head turn, and so forth). Both the interpreting radiologist and SLP render separate reports on their respective findings; 92611 motion fluoroscopic evaluation of swallowing function by cine recording or video recording represents the comprehensive evaluation of swallowing by the SLP when performed with a radiologist, who in turn reports 74230 for radiological supervision and interpretation.

Generally, otolaryngologists do not perform these studies and, if performed and interpreted by others, they cannot bill for these services. If the studies are reviewed by an otolaryngologist, this work should be documented in the E/M service as part of the medical decision making.

Speech and swallowing therapy if done by qualified speech therapist may be reported with the following:

Procedure	Code(s)	Notes
Speech and swallowing therapy codes	92610	Evaluation of oral and pharyngeal swallowing function represents a clinical (nonradiologic) evaluation of a patient's oral–motor, laryngeal, and swallowing function with a continuum of liquid and solid boluses, including introduction of compensatory strategies.
	92526	Treatment of swallowing dysfunction and/or oral function for feeding typically is used for the SLP's work with patients undergoing swallowing therapy.
	92520	Laryngeal function studies (ie, aerodynamic testing and acoustic testing) may be used to report measurements of airflow and acoustic characteristics (eg, jitter and shimmer).

These codes should not be reported by the physician using incident-to billing. They may be reported using the NPI of the SLP, depending on payer rules.

Transnasal esophagoscopy may be used in the office setting to help evaluate swallowing as well as anatomic abnormalities. It is distinct from transoral flexible esophagoscopy (most frequently performed by gastroenterologists) and rigid esophagoscopy (typically performed under general anesthesia and not in the office) and is represented by a code family of 2: diagnostic and with biopsy. If performed with other upper aerodigestive endoscopy, transnasal esophagoscopy may be reported separately with modifier 59, if a separate endoscope is used and ideally for a different, well-documented diagnosis. Be sure to be familiar with state regulations and payer requirements regarding submission of photographs and/or videos. The pertinent codes are as follows:

| Transnasal esophagoscopy | 43197 | Esophagoscopy, flexible, transnasal; diagnostic, including collection of specimen(s) by brushing or washing, when performed (separate procedure) |
| | 43198 | Esophagoscopy, flexible, transnasal; with biopsy, single or multiple |

REFERENCES

1. Ahlman, et al, editors. CPT® professional edition. Chicago: American Medical Assocation; 2019.
2. CPT® Assistant. Chicago: American Medical Assocation; 2016.

FURTHER READINGS

AMA CPT® Network. Available at: https://www.ama-assn.org/amaone/cpt-current-procedural-terminology.
CPT® for ENT-AAO/HNS. Available at: https://www.entnet.org/content/CPT-ents.

Surgical Cosmetic Procedures of the Face

Lara Devgan, MD, MPH[a,b,*], Priyanka Singh[a,c], Kamala Durairaj[a,d]

KEYWORDS

- Plastic surgery • Facelift • Blepharoplasty • Rhinoplasty • Necklift • Neurotoxins
- Dermal fillers

KEY POINTS

- Surgical procedures can address the upper, middle, and lower face through the following: brow lift, blepharoplasty, rhinoplasty, lip lift, facelift, necklift, and submental liposuction.
- The surgical techniques and procedures described are the gold standard to help enhance facial beauty, optimize facial features, and achieve antiaging or facial rejuvenation goals.
- For each individual, the optimal strategy to achieving youthful facial beauty varies depending on health, lifestyle, time limitations, amount of change desired, and the willingness to participate in surgery.

INTRODUCTION

Surgical facial rejuvenation embodies an extensive spectrum of procedures aimed at enhancing beauty and reversing aging-related changes to the face. Age-related concerns include descent of the brows, tissue laxity and hollowing of the periorbita, malar descent causing heaviness of the nasolabial folds and jowls, blunting of the jawline, laxity of the neck, and weakening of the substructural muscular tissues of the head and neck, the submuscular aponeurotic system and platysma.[1] Non–age-related concerns encompass issues related to optimization of facial features, including the aesthetic undesirability of the nose, lips, and facial proportions.[2] Surgery, considered the gold standard for facial rejuvenation, allows for the removal of excess skin, suture plication of tissue descent, and manual reshaping to more powerfully restore the upper face, midface, and lower face.[3]

That being said, surgical procedures do have limitations. They do not serve as a treatment for fine lines, sun damage, irregular pigmentation, or textural issues, which

Disclosure Statement: The authors have nothing to disclose.
[a] PLLC Plastic & Reconstructive Surgery, 969 Park Avenue, New York, NY 10028, USA; [b] American Board of Plastic Surgery; [c] Princeton University, Princeton, NJ, USA; [d] Georgetown University, Washington, DC, USA
* Corresponding author. 969 Park Avenue, New York, NY 10028.
E-mail address: info@laradevganmd.com

Otolaryngol Clin N Am 52 (2019) 425–441
https://doi.org/10.1016/j.otc.2019.02.001
0030-6665/19/© 2019 Elsevier Inc. All rights reserved.

are better addressed with resurfacing techniques. Surgery requires a longer amount of recovery time and increased discomfort compared with minimally invasive interventions.[3,4] Additionally, because an incision is necessary in the completion of facial surgical procedures, surgical procedures do create scars, although they can often be camouflaged or hidden with proper technique.[3,4] An appropriate treatment plan must be determined in consultation with the operating surgeon to weigh a variety of factors, including age, desired end results, goals and expectations with regard to recovery and downtime, and medical comorbidities.[3,4] The goal of this article is to provide a general overview of the following surgical procedures: brow lift, blepharoplasty, rhinoplasty, lip lift, rhytidectomy, lower rhytidectomy (neck lift), and submental liposuction. All surgical procedures are performed in an accredited operating room.

UPPER FACE
Brow Lift

Progressive descent of the brows can create a tired, stern, or angry impression on the resting face. Brow lifting, a widely performed cosmetic procedure, aims at generating a normal resting impression by addressing forehead rhytids, frown muscle imbalance, upper eyelid aesthetics, lateral temporal laxity, and abnormal expression.[5–7] According to the American Society of Plastic Surgeons, 39,886 brow lifts were performed in 2017.[8]

Technique

The brow lift is performed under intravenous sedation under the supervision of a board-certified anesthesiologist. Critical anatomic landmarks during the brow lift include the sentinel vein, the path of the frontal branch of the facial nerve, the temporalis muscle, and the location of the supraorbital and supratrochlear nerves.[5] Avoidance of excessive upward traction and cautery in this region during dissection decreases the risk of injury to the nerve branches.[5]

Endoscopic brow lifting is a preferred, less invasive method of brow lifting. Benefits include less scarring and less edema. The approach remains challenging, however, in patients with a high hairline or acutely sloped forehead. This technique often requires access incisions that are placed directly posterior to the hairline to maximize traction on the scalp and forehead.[5]

During lateral brow lifting, the scalp flap is retracted superolaterally with an Allis clamp and the excess is excised to achieve redraping of the lateral orbital region. The scalp is secured to the deep temporal fascia with a 3-0 polydioxanone suture and the skin is closed with surgical staples.[5] Possible risk includes eyebrow or forehead scar and persistence of forehead wrinkles, which can be camouflaged in the patients' rhytides and diminished by the conjoint use of botulinum toxin, respectively.[6]

Practitioners have found high levels of patient satisfaction with the brow lift procedure. Eighty-four percent of patients stated that they would undergo the procedure again.[9] Although the surgery itself is more time consuming than alternatives such as neurotoxin-mediated brow lifting and suture-based thread lifting, the procedure is considered the gold standard with the best ability to produce sustainable elevation of the forehead and brow region.

Blepharoplasty The eye plays an essential role in facial aesthetics. Blepharoplasty, a procedure to repair or reconstruct of the eyelid, can help to generate facial harmony and decrease the perception of aging by addressing tired-looking eyes, skin laxity, or droopy eyelids. In combination with other facial and skin rejuvenation procedures including the brow or midface lift, it can also restore an overall youthful impression.[10] Blepharoplasty is the third most commonly performed aesthetic surgical procedure in the United States, after liposuction and breast augmentation.[11] More than 200,000 blepharoplasty procedures were conducted in 2017.[8]

Upper eyelid blepharoplasty

The American Society of Ophthalmic Plastic and Reconstructive Surgery members perform, on average, 196 upper eyelid procedures per year.[8]

Technique The chief element to upper blepharoplasty is the cautious removal of excess preaponeurotic fat. The patient is marked in an upright seated position to plan an incision in the natural lid crease, with a lenticular or crescent-shaped skin excision planned, with attention to both symmetry and preservation of sufficient upper lid height. Fat excision focuses on decreasing herniation of the medial fat pad and is minimized in the middle third of the lid to avoid an A-frame deformity from overresection. The upper eyelid blepharoplasty can be performed under local anesthesia with the patient conscious.

Excess brow fat pad and internal browpexy can be performed by suturing the dermis of the brow to the periosteum at the desired peak of the brow with 4-0 Prolene. Transpalpebral resection of the corrugator can be performed safely by dissecting just posterior to the orbicularis in the nasal portion of the upper lid until the corrugator is identified.[5] The corrugator should be removed from medial to supratrochlear nerve and just lateral to the supraorbital nerve. In select cases, supratarsal fixation may be performed with 6-0 Vicryl suturing of the levator aponeurosis to the dermal lid crease to preserve the upper lid crease and minimize the risk of postblepharoplasty ptosis.[5] The skin is closed with a fine nonabsorbable suture, such as continuous 6-0 nylon.

Lower eyelid blepharoplasty

Aging induces changes in the lower eyelid, including excess orbital septum laxity, herniation of the crow's feet, orbital fat, and periocular wrinkles.[12] On average, the American Society of Ophthalmic Plastic and Reconstructive Surgery members perform 46 lower eyelid procedures per year.[8]

Contemporary aesthetic trends in lower eyelid blepharoplasty focus on reducing eye bag prominence while contributing to the smooth, youthful transition of the lower eyelid–cheek interface. This technique requires preserving and enhancing the eyelid volume. More conservative skin excision, orbicularis muscle preservation, and supportive canthal suspension have become critical constituents of lower eyelid surgery.[13]

Technique The lower eyelid blepharoplasty is performed under intravenous sedation under the supervision of a board-certified anesthesiologist. In younger patients who have no demonstrable lid laxity, transconjunctival blepharoplasty is effective to excise or redrape fat.[5] In patients with excess lower lid skin and periorbital aging, this author prefers a transconjunctival approach to lower lid fat pads, followed by a transcutaneous skin pinch excision. Combined with lateral canthal anchoring in select cases, optimal control of lid position and lower lid aging changes can be achieved.[5]

Lateral canthal anchoring is recommended in patients with lid laxity because it provides lower lid support, thus controlling lid shape and minimizing the risk of lid malposition.[5] A 5-mm incision is made just lateral to the lateral canthus. The skin is dissected from the pretarsal muscle from a lateral to medial direction. A stairstep incision is made in the inferior orbicularis muscle, preserving 4 to 5 mm of pretarsal orbicularis. The skin muscle flap is dissected inferiorly in the preperiosteal plane to release the orbitomalar ligament. A double-armed 4-0 Mersilene suture is used to join the tarsal plate of the lateral canthus to the orbital rim at the level of the pupil. This lid should follow the curve of the globe. The skin and muscle are tightened superolaterally, separate from the canthal anchoring, to allow for aesthetic tightening of the skin and muscle underneath the lid. The muscle is sutured with a 4-0 Vicryl 3-point quilting suture to the temporal fascia and lateral orbital rim periosteum. The skin is excised conservatively along the subciliary margin and closed with a 5-0 fast absorbing gut suture. The 5-mm lateral incision is closed with interrupted or running sutures.[5,13]

Alternatives for lower eyelid rejuvenation include fillers and skin resurfacing, generally less complex procedures. The practitioner and patient should choose the best approach to address the concerns and produce the desired outcome.[14]

Concluding Remarks Blepharoplasty procedures have the ability to decrease age-related changes to the periorbital region. The blepharoplasty office procedure is

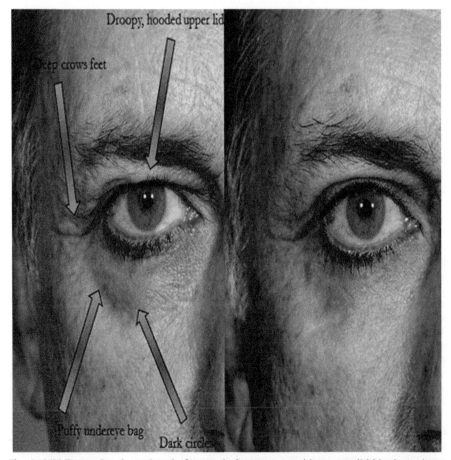

Fig. 1. Middle-aged male patient before and after upper and lower eyelid blepharoplasty. Notice an improvement in the hooding of the upper lid and a decreased appearance of crows feet, dark circles, and puffiness under the eye.

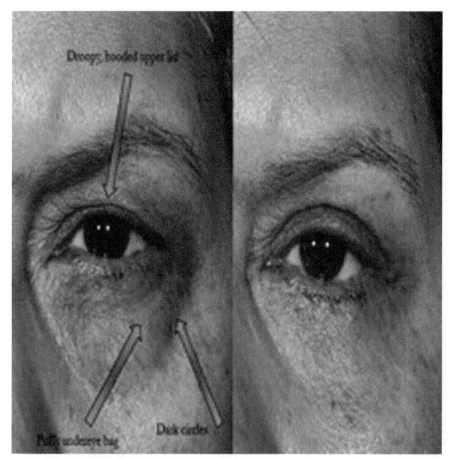

Fig. 2. Elderly male patient before and after upper and lower eyelid blepharoplasty. Notice an improvement in dark circles, puffiness under the eyes, and hooding of the upper eyelid.

safe, effective, and well-accepted by patients. In a blepharoplasty satisfaction survey conducted in 2008%, 97% of patients said they would refer family and friends to undergo eyelid surgery in the office.[12] Patients enjoy the cost savings and decreased anesthetic risk as compared with the same procedure performed under intravenous or general anesthesia. Risks include overresection, eyelid malposition, alteration in shape of the eyes, undesirable scarring, and retrobulbar hematoma, which requires immediate intervention to preserve vision. Precision and attention to detail are needed to reduce these risks (**Figs. 1–3**).

MIDFACE
Rhinoplasty

Rhinoplasty surgery aims to provide desirable nasal features and optimization of the nose by improving facial harmony. The third most common cosmetic surgical procedure in 2017 according to the American Society of Plastic Surgeons, 218,924 rhinoplasty procedures were performed.[8] Rhinoplasty surgery is an effective option to address midface irregularities and create an aesthetically pleasing facial balance.

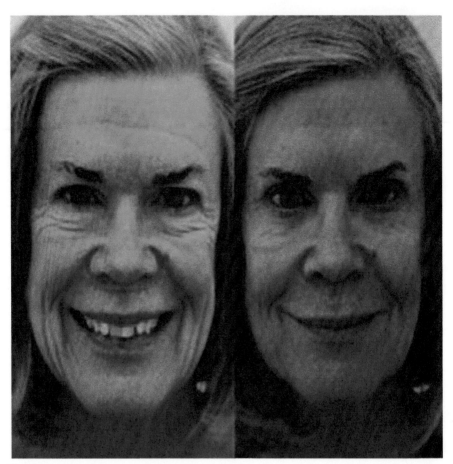

Fig. 3. Middle-aged female patient before and after upper and lower eyelid blepharoplasty. Notice an improvement in the hooding of the upper eyelid, and a decrease in appearance of crows feet and excess skin under the eyes.

Chin augmentation is often performed in conjunction with rhinoplasty to improve overall facial aesthetics.

Technique

This author uses both open and closed rhinoplasty techniques, depending on patient concerns and anatomic features needing correction, although our preference is for the closed approach owing to the decreased tissue trauma and improved recovery. The surgical rhinoplasty is performed under intravenous sedation under the supervision of a board-certified anesthesiologist.

Dorsum A dorsal hump reduction can be performed as either a composite or component reduction. The latter allows for the selective reduction of the septum proper and modification of the upper lateral cartilages as needed.[14] This technique can prevent an inverted-V deformity, internal nasal valve dysfunction, and atypical dorsal aesthetic lines. Reconstitution of the septum can be performed with upper lateral cartilage tension spanning sutures, spreader grafts, or autospreader

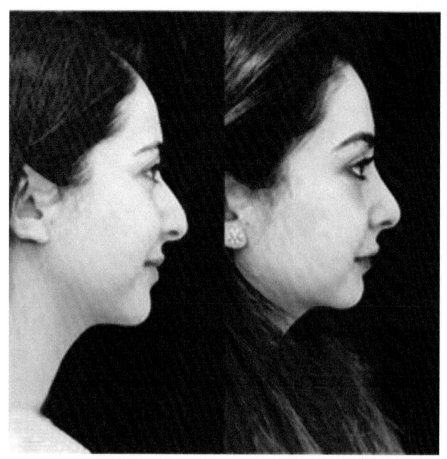

Fig. 4. Before and after: surgical rhinoplasty.

flaps. Autospreader flaps or spreader grafts are best suited to reconstruct a narrowed midvault, correct the deviated nose, or treat internal nasal valve dysfunction.[15]

Septum Septal deviation can lead to nasal obstruction and/or external nasal deviation. Deviation includes a septal tilt, anteroposterior deviation, craniocaudal deviation, or septal spurs. Septoplasty can be used to correct the deviation as well as harvest cartilage to be used for grafting.[15] During standard septoplasty, mucoperichondrial and mucoperiosteal flaps are elevated. The deviated or deformed intervening cartilage and bone are removed or repositioned to the midline. When removing cartilage, the surgeon should preserve a 15-mm-wide dorsal and caudal L-strut. This process can be difficult in caudal septal deviations.[15]

Tip The first step of tip refinement is assessment of tip rotation and projection. Alteration of these 2 elements can be performed via cephalic trim, tip suturing, cartilage grafting, or a combination of these techniques.[15] The lower lateral cartilage is separated from the upper lateral cartilage at the scroll area. Cephalic trim can be used to decrease vertical height of the lateral crura. Ultimately, 8 to

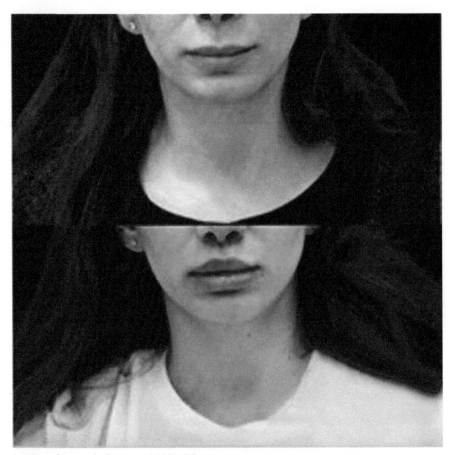

Fig. 5. Before and after: surgical lip lift.

10 mm medially and 5 to 7 mm laterally of the lateral crura should remain. Cephalic trim decreases supratip fullness. The supratip break represents a subtle shadow in the supratip area, where the more posteriorly positioned dorsum transitions to the anteriorly located tip. Cephalic trim can reposition the supratip break more inferiorly and consequently refine the nasal tip.[15] Excessive cephalic trim will result in alar deformities or external nasal valve dysfunction. The interdomal suture is a useful technique to place between the domal segments of the middle crura of the lower lateral cartilages. The sutures can increase tip projection, decrease the angle of domal divergence, narrow the tip-defining points, and refine the infratip lobule.[15]

Osteotomies Nasal osteotomies close open roof deformities, decrease nasal bony width, and straighten the deviated nasal pyramid.[15] The goal is a pleasing contour and narrowed, more refined nasal appearance.

Concluding remarks
In a study exploring long-term patient satisfaction after rhinoplasty, 88% experienced a significant improvement after rhinoplasty.[3] Satisfaction was unrelated to the open or

closed technique used for revision.[16] Rhinoplasty can enhance facial harmony via correction of the nasal features, if performed with a thorough facial anatomic knowledge and an understanding of the patient's desired outcome.

Risks of rhinoplasty include epistaxis, infection, scarring, asymmetry, difficulty breathing as a result of internal or external nasal valve collapse, and the need for revision. This author prefers a conservative approach to rhinoplasty, which minimizes tissue resection and favors reshaping techniques, in an effort to preserve long-term function and stability, as well as minimize these risks (**Fig. 4**).

Lip Lift

Beautification of the lips also contributes to midface harmony. Recently, fuller lips have emerged as a desirable trait. With age, lips become thinner, invert, and show redundancy.[15,17] The aim of lip lift surgery is to improve the vertical height of the upper lip and decrease an elongated philtral distance.[18] Although dermal fillers are popular for injectable lip augmentation, surgical upper lip lift is thought to produce the most definitive and permanent results.

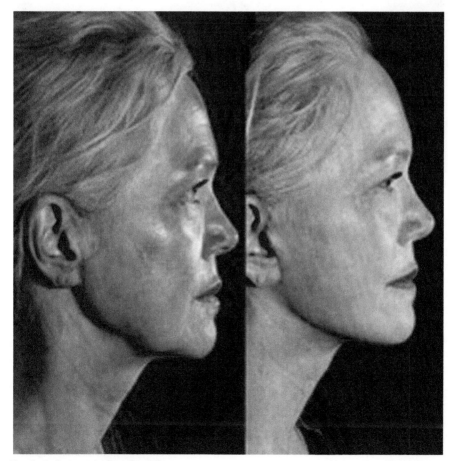

Fig. 6. Before and after: facelift.

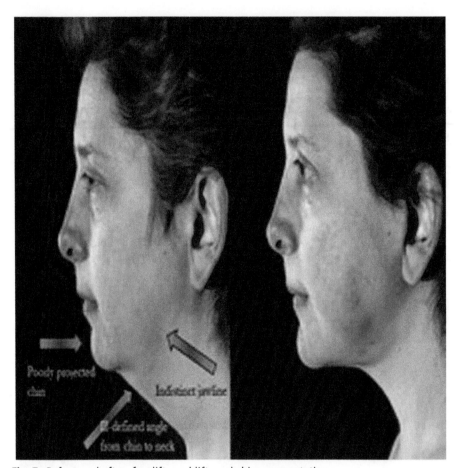

Fig. 7. Before and after: facelift, necklift, and chin augmentation.

Technique

Key anatomic points, including the philtral distance and base of the columella, are marked. The lip lift procedure can be performed under local anesthesia alone with the patient awake. This author prefers a modified approach to minimize incision length and avoid trauma to the orbicularis oris. An incision is made from the midpoint of the base of columella and is extended into the perialar region, medial to the nasolabial area.[16] A skin excision is marked in a bullhorn-shaped pattern to provide for an ideal philtral distance of 11 to 13 mm. Then, the subcutaneous tissue is dissected and debulked up to the vermilion, without compromising the orbicularis oris muscle.[18,19] The lip incision is then repaired in layers.

Concluding remarks

Patient satisfaction with the lip lift procedure is high, because the results are permanent and the future need for filler is decreased.[19] The procedure produces a more youthful look with fuller lips and decreased philtral distance. Risks include scarring and asymmetry, both of which can be mitigated by careful surgical planning and execution (**Fig. 5**).

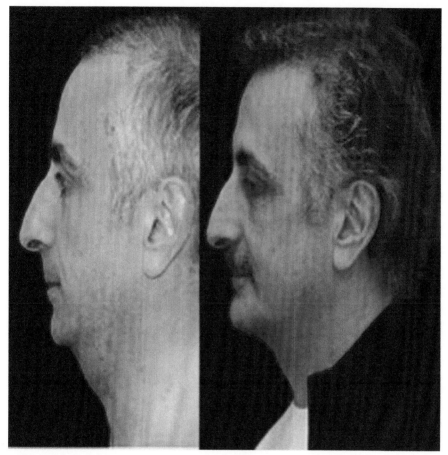

Fig. 8. Before and after: chin augmentation, necklift, and blepharoplasty.

LOWER FACE
Face Lift/Neck Lift

A facelift is a surgical technique that restores youthful bone structure to the jaw, cheeks, and neck. The focus is placed on resuspending the muscular substructure of the face and neck (the superficial musculoaponeurotic system [SMAS] and platysma) to achieve lasting results. Facelift surgery is 1 of the top 5 most commonly performed plastic surgical procedures in America, with many patients interested in rejuvenating their middle and lower face and neck appearance. More than125,000 face lift procedures and more than 50,000 neck lift procedures were performed in 2017.[8]

Technique

The facelift is performed under intravenous sedation under the supervision of a board-certified anesthesiologist. There are 5 layers to consider when performing a face lift: skin, subcutaneous fat, the SMAS muscle layer, a thin layer of transparent fascia, and the branches of the facial nerve. The SMAS layer contains many of the muscles of facial expression: frontalis, orbicularis oculi, zygomaticus major and minor, and platysma.[11]

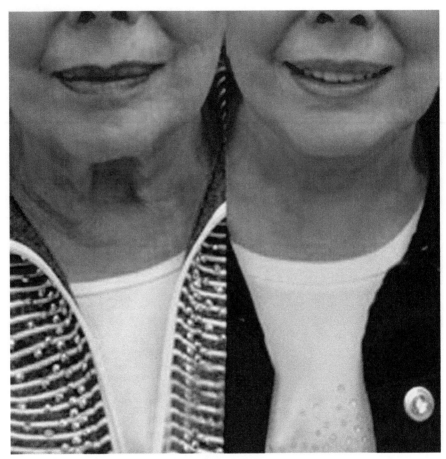

Fig. 9. Before and after: necklift and facelift.

The procedure can be performed in the subcutaneous plane, the sub-SMAS (deep) plane, the subperiosteal plane, or a combination of these planes. The subcutaneous lift is one of the first forms of face lifting and has been described as discontinuous ellipsoidal skin excisions in natural skin creases.[19] However, standalone subcutaneous lifts are limited in their ability to reposition deep tissues. Sub-SMAS dissection, in contrast, yields a thicker and more robust composite flap with longer lasting results made possible by deeper dissection.[20]

This author prefers SMAS plication or resection to achieve more durable results than a subcutaneous-only facelift, but to decrease the risks of a deep plane technique. SMAS dissection involves a transverse incision in the SMAS just below the zygomatic arch and an intersecting preauricular SMAS incision that extends over the angle of the mandible and along the anterior border of the sternomastoid muscle. The SMAS is elevated off the parotid fascia in continuity with the platysma muscle in the neck. The dissection endpoint is just beyond the anterior border of the parotid gland. The SMAS–platysma flap is rotated in a cephaloposterior direction, trimmed, and sutured to the immobile SMAS along the original incision lines. A

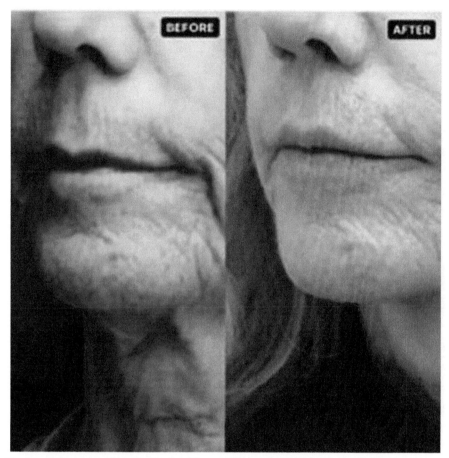

Fig. 10. Before and after: lip lift, facelift, necklift, and erbium laser resurfacing.

strip of SMAS is excised on an oblique line between the angle of the mandible and lateral canthus. The SMASectomy procedure is the most frequently performed facelift technique in the United States today. This technique has major advantages; it can be individualized to different face shapes and achieves powerful results with limited risks.[11]

For desirable results, anterior adjustment of the platysma is crucial. The subplatysma fat pocket, if present in a heavy neck, must be excised. For patients who are not candidates for an upward lift, a posterior submental incision and a more radical submental lipectomy with a platysma sling (submental neck lift) is helpful. Cutting the platysma, fashioning the sling, and defatting can increase the duration of the lift effect, but this can only be determined with a long-term follow-up.[21]

Concluding Remarks

The risks of facelift and necklift include hematoma, facial nerve injury, skin necrosis, and undesirable scarring. A modern approach to facelift that favors modest skin pulling and more meaningful substructural elevation can minimize these risks and also

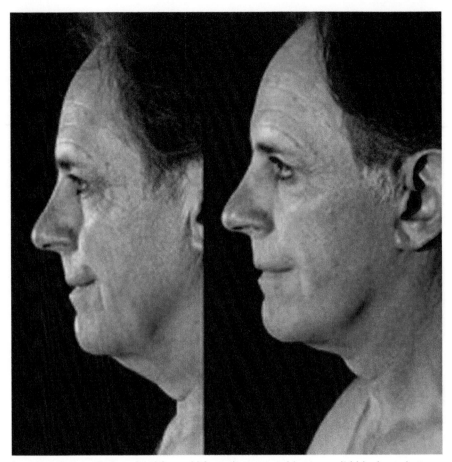

Fig. 11. Before and after: facelift, necklift, and upper and lower eyelid blepharoplasty.

attain more natural-looking results. There are no other techniques that are as powerful as the face lift or neck left in addressing midface descent, neck laxity, excess skin, and jowling (**Figs. 6–11**).

Submental Liposuction

The young, aesthetically pleasing face is wider at the cheeks and narrow at the chin. With age and weight gain, individuals develop unwanted fat deposition. A double chin can develop and the jawline loses its contour.

Although facelift and neck lift are considered the gold standard procedures for addressing facial aging, for younger patients and those who would like a shortened recovery with fewer incisions, submental liposuction is a viable option. Submental liposuction is a minimally invasive contouring procedure for the lower face. Using 1 to 3 tiny 0.5-cm incisions placed in inconspicuous locations, submental liposuction allows for the slimming and reshaping of the chin region by removing excess fat deposits.[8] The procedure can help to improve the neck–chin contour line.

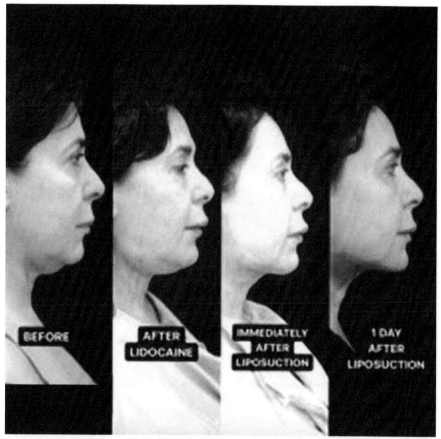

Fig. 12. Middle-aged female patient before and after submental liposuction. Notice the decrease in submental fullness and a defined jawline immediately after and 1 day after.

Technique

Submental liposuction can be performed under local anesthesia in the awake patient. A small, 5-mm incision should be placed in the submental skin crease. The patient should be marked bilaterally at the angle of the mandible and at the anticipated position of the marginal mandibular nerve.[20] A 3-mm liposuction cannula is then introduced without suction. A fanning technique can be used to break down adhesions and scarred tissue in the target area. Then, suction is applied to the cannula to remove fat. At the end of the procedure, the treatment area is inspected to ensure a symmetric result.[20]

Concluding remarks

The most common complications that come with submental liposuction is contour irregularity, including notching, divots, and an irregular appearance of the skin. Another complication is injury to the surrounding structures of the neck, specifically the marginal mandibular branch of the facial nerve.[21] This complication can be mitigated by cautious suctioning in the region of the nerve and continuous checks of symmetry (**Figs. 12** and **13**).

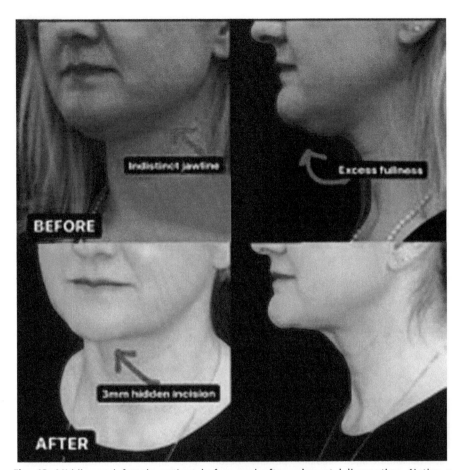

Fig. 13. Middle-aged female patient before and after submental liposuction. Notice a decrease in submental fullness and a defined jawline.

SUMMARY

For each individual, the optimal strategy to achieving youthful facial beauty will vary depending on health, lifestyle, time limitations, amount of change desired, and willingness to participate in surgery. Surgery is thought to produce the most permanent and best result; with the utmost attention to detail, an artistic eye, and genuine care, office-based cosmetic surgery can produce natural results including rejuvenated facial features.

REFERENCES

1. Tardy E. Facial aesthetic surgery. Plast Reconstr Surg 1995;96(6):1477.
2. Chuang J. Overview of facial plastic surgery and current developments. Surg J (N Y) 2016. https://doi.org/10.1055/s-0036-1572360.
3. Hellings PW, Trenité GJN. Long-term patient satisfaction after revision rhinoplasty. Laryngoscope 2007;117(6):985–9.
4. Monheit G. Neurotoxins. Plastic and Reconstructive Surgery 2015;136. https://doi.org/10.1097/prs.0000000000001771.

5. Codner MA, Kikkawa DO, Korn BS, et al. Blepharoplasty and brow lift. Plast Reconstr Surg 2010;126(1). https://doi.org/10.1097/prs.0b013e3181dbc4a2.

6. Hernandez OP, Bracchini JM. Management of the heavy brows: long-term surgical options. Facial Plast Surg 2018;34(01):036–42.

7. Paul MD. The evolution of the brow lift in aesthetic plastic surgery. Plast Reconstr Surg 2001;108(5):1409–22.

8. American Society of Plastic Surgeons. Available at: https://www.plasticsurgery.org/reconstructive-procedures. Accessed June 12, 2018.

9. Booth AJ. The direct brow lift: efficacy, complications, and patient satisfaction. Br J Ophthalmol 2004;88(5):688–91.

10. Naik M, Honavar S, Das S, et al. Blepharoplasty: an overview. J Cutan Aesthet Surg 2009;2(1):6.

11. Kossler AL, Peng GL, Yoo DB, et al. Current trends in upper and lower eyelid blepharoplasty among American Society of Ophthalmic Plastic and Reconstructive Surgery members. Ophthalmic Plast Reconstr Surg 2017;1. https://doi.org/10.1097/iop.0000000000000849.

12. Harley DH, Collins DR. Patient satisfaction after blepharoplasty performed as office surgery using oral medication with the patient under local anesthesia. Aesthetic Plast Surg 2007;32(1):77–81.

13. Thorne C, Chung KC, Gosain A, et al. Grabb and Smith's plastic surgery. Philadelphia: Wolters Kluwer/Lippincott Williams & Wilkins Health; 2014.

14. Tanna N, Nguyen KT, Ghavami A, et al. Evidence-based medicine. Plast Reconstr Surg 2018;141(1). https://doi.org/10.1097/prs.0000000000003977.

15. Segall L, Ellis DA. Therapeutic options for lip augmentation. Facial Plast Surg Clin North Am 2007;15(4):485–90.

16. Loghmani S, Momeni A, Eidy M. Results of a unilateral lip lift for correction of a vertical disproportion in upper lip vascular anomalies. Indian J Plast Surg 2009;42(1):13.

17. Fanous N. Correction of thin lips. Plast Reconstr Surg 1984;74(1):33–41.

18. Bellinga RJ, Capitán L, Simon D, et al. Technical and clinical considerations for facial feminization surgery with rhinoplasty and related procedures. JAMA Facial Plast Surg 2017;19(3):175.

19. Wan D, Small KH, Barton FE. Face lift. Plast Reconstr Surg 2015;136(5). https://doi.org/10.1097/prs.0000000000001695.

20. Alamoudi U, Taylor B, Mackay C, et al. Submental liposuction for the management of lymphedema following head and neck cancer treatment: a randomized controlled trial. J Otolaryngol Head Neck Surg 2018;47(1). https://doi.org/10.1186/s40463-018-0263-1.

21. Ellenbogen R, Karlin JV. Visual criteria for success in restoring the youthful neck. Plast Reconstr Surg 1980;66(6):826–37.

Minimally Invasive Facial Cosmetic Procedures

Lara Devgan, MD, MPH[a,b,*], Priyanka Singh[a,c], Kamala Durairaj[a,d]

KEYWORDS

- Plastic surgery • Nonsurgical • Rhinoplasty • Neurotoxins • Dermal fillers

KEY POINTS

- Nonsurgical cosmetic facial procedures restore a youthful appearance by enhancing features of symmetry, contour, and positive expression.
- Injectables, including neurotoxins and dermal fillers, can reduce facial wrinkles and skin texture changes caused by aging.
- Deoxycholic acid is used for minimally invasive fat contouring to improve the jawline and chin.
- Lasers, chemical peels, and microneedling are effective skin resurfacing techniques.
- The techniques and procedures described are used to help enhance facial beauty, optimize facial features, and achieve antiaging or facial rejuvenation goals.

INTRODUCTION

Facial optimization is accomplished through the use of minimally invasive cosmetic procedures including injectable and skin resurfacing techniques via the use of toxins, dermal fillers, biomaterials, lasers, and other skin resurfacing devices to improve outcomes.[1] Less invasive than surgery, injectables and skin resurfacing techniques target various facial irregularities including wrinkles and fine lines, decrease in volume and contour, and unwanted fat. Determining the best approach for a given patient involves careful consideration of the patient's health conditions, unique anatomic characteristics, tissue quality, and desired results. Collectively, these procedures aim to optimize facial aesthetics by creating a youthful appearance, enhancing symmetry, augmenting facial contours, and improving proportions of the face and neck.

This article broadly address the spectrum of nonsurgical cosmetic procedures to rejuvenate and optimize the face. Nonsurgical injectable procedures include the use

Disclosure Statement: The authors have nothing to disclose.
[a] PLLC Plastic & Reconstructive Surgery, 969 Park Ave Suite 1G New York, NY 10028, USA;
[b] American Board of Plastic Surgery; [c] Princeton University, Princeton, NJ, USA; [d] Georgetown University, Washington, DC, USA
* Corresponding author. 969 Park Avenue, New York, NY 10028.
E-mail address: info@laradevganmd.com

of neurotoxin, dermal fillers, and deoxycholic acid, whereas skin resurfacing techniques include lasers, chemical peels, and microneedling.

INJECTABLES

Less invasive than surgery, injectables target various facial irregularities including wrinkles and fine lines, decrease in volume and contour, and unwanted fat. Neurotoxin injections are used to address fine lines and wrinkles; dermal fillers to restore a youthful facial impression and volume; and deoxycholic acid to dissolve fat in unwanted areas, primarily submentally. Injectables are an optimal procedure for those who are in search of minimally invasive therapy for treating facial aging, because they have minimal associated downtime and recovery.

Neurotoxins

Facial aging is marked by skin texture changes and wrinkle formation caused by movement of the underlying facial muscles. Injection of botulin neurotoxin is a widely used therapy to treat and prevent wrinkle formation on the face and neck. Since its discovery as a wrinkle minimizer, botulinum toxin injection is the leading male and female minimally invasive cosmetic procedure in the United States, with 7.2 million procedures performed in 2017 alone.[2–4]

Technique
The botulinum toxin type A, the most potent type of botulinum neurotoxins in humans, works by inhibiting the release of acetylcholine, a neurotransmitter found at the neuromuscular junction of striated muscle fibers. This results in denervation of the muscle and consequently, temporarily diminished muscle activity. Botulinum toxins take 2 to 4 days postinjection to weaken muscle action and 7 to 10 days to reach maximal muscle denervation. The effect is temporary because nerve endings form "peripheral sprouts" with time.[5]

Upper face The most common area for botulinum toxin treatment is the upper face, which includes the glabella, forehead, brows, and crow's feet.[4] For the glabella and forehead regions, the goal of treatment is to soften undesirable lines without eliminating expressiveness.[4] A commonly used strategy is to place the injection line parallel and inferior to the deep furrow crossing the middle to upper third of the forehead.[4]

Periorbital lines or crow's feet, one of the earliest signs of aging, are typically treated with three equal injections of 2 to 4 U Botox evenly spaced along an arc lying at least 1 cm external to the orbital rim to avoid diffusion to the palpebral portion of the orbicularis oculi or to the levator palpebrae muscle.[4] The middle injection is to be aligned with the lateral canthus. Injections flanking this point at 8 to 10 mm are then placed, but their exact sites depend on the width of the patient's canthal lines (**Fig. 1**).

Lower face Lower face botulinum toxin treatment includes targeted therapy for the depressor anguli oris, orbicularis oris, masseter muscles, and mentalis.

Treatment of the orbicularis oris can attain temporary improvement of hyperdynamic vertical perioral rhytides. Total dosages range between 4 and 5 U of Botox. One-unit aliquots are delivered over four injection points along the superior vermilion border. Two injection points are used on the lower vermilion order 1 cm medial from the oral commissure to prevent unwanted spread into muscles and inserting into the modiolus.[6]

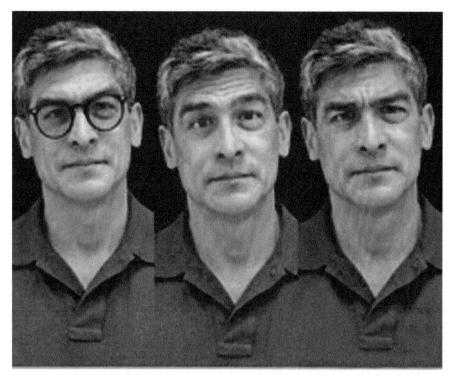

Fig. 1. Upper face target areas for cosmetic neurotoxin injection (forehead, glabella, crow's feet).

The mentalis muscle serves to elevate the skin of the chin and its fibers intermingle with the orbicularis oris and depressor labii inferioris. A hyperactive mentalis muscle can lead to wrinkling and creasing of the mental area. Smoothing of these wrinkles is achieved with the injection of either 2 U of toxin into each belly of the muscle, staying close to the midline spread to the depressor labii inferioris, or 4 U of toxin directly into the insertion point of both bellies of the mentalis muscle centrally on the mandible. It is also crucial to place injections deep to avoid the more superficial depressor labii inferioris.[6]

An overactive masseter conveys squaring of the lower face, an aesthetically displeasing and masculinizing feature, particularly in women. Previous work supports the use of Botox in the reduction of unwanted masseteric hypertrophy. Palpate the point of maximal muscle hypertrophy on clenching along the mandibular order and mark this as the primary injection point to optimize safety.[6]

Concluding remarks

Botulinum toxin has become the gold standard minimally invasive facial rejuvenation[5]; Botox, Dysport, Xeomin, or other related neurotoxins are an effective method to soften wrinkles and fine lines for all areas of the face. With an individualized approach to satisfy a patient's desired outcomes, neurotoxin-related procedures have yielded high patient satisfaction regarding facial and age appearance.[7] However, toxins only address muscle-controlled wrinkles and lines. Fine etched lines and those caused by photodamage do not improve solely with neurotoxin, a factor that should be taken into consideration when developing a treatment plan.[5]

Dermal Fillers

Dermal fillers combat facial aging with volume restoration. As more individuals opt for noninvasive aesthetic rejuvenation, demand for injectable dermal fillers continues to grow.[2] In the past 5 years, dermal filler treatments have increased by 35%.[8] Fillers are injected to restore volume lost because of age or disease, provide facial contour, and help maintain a youthful appearance.[9] The most commonly used fillers are based on hyaluronic acid, although biostimulatory products, such as calcium hydroxyapatite (Radiesse) and poly-L-lactic acid (Sculptra), are also popular and powerful options.

Traditionally, these anatomic changes caused by aging were corrected via surgical modalities, and the surgical facelift will remain the gold standard for addressing lax and aged facial skin.[5] However, hyaluronic acid fillers have more recently found a niche in volumetric restoration. For candidates who are unwilling to undergo elective aesthetic surgery, dermal filler therapies offer a viable treatment option to restore facial youth.[5]

Technique

The area of injection and the surrounding skin should be cleaned properly. Anesthesia is provided with topical lidocaine cream application of regional nerve blocks. The choice of injection technique depends on the location, its indication, the type of filler, and needle size.[10] The techniques include: linear threading technique, serial puncture, fanning, cross-hatching, depot, fern, and cone. The first four are used commonly and the last three are only used in specific situations. It is crucial to place the filler in the right location and the bevel orientation should not pose a significant issue at any site.[8]

It takes 2 to 3 weeks for full results of dermal fillers to become apparent, and the effects last anywhere between 3 months and 2 years. The duration depends on the type of filler used, where on the patient's face it was injected, how expressive the face is, and the patient's metabolic rate.[8] After repeated use of dermal fillers, many patients find that they have results that last longer than expected because hyaluronic acid (collagen)-based dermal fillers stimulate the body's own collagen supply.[8] Patients are advised to avoid strenuous exercise on the day of treatment, to avoid drinking excessive alcohol within 2 days of treatment, and to sleep with their head elevated (**Figs. 2–11**).

Concluding remarks

Fillers have revolutionized the approach to facial augmentation because of their long-lasting correction with fewer side effects, greater lift, and the possibility of reversing unwanted aesthetic results.[11] As patients lean toward minimally invasive alternatives, dermal facial fillers continue to gain popularity.

Deoxycholic Acid

Deoxycholic acid (Kybella/Kythera), another injectable therapy, aims to permanently dissolve fat in target areas. A recent survey conducted by the American Society for Dermatologic Surgery demonstrated that 67% of respondents were unsatisfied by excess fat under the chin/neck.[12] Submental fullness creates an older and heavier impression, and reduction of fat in the area can not only create a more youthful impression but also improve the contour of the jawline and chin. Kybella, a Food and Drug Administration–approved injectable deoxycholic acid treatment, has been introduced as a noninvasive option that destroys fat cells, specifically in the submental region.[10]

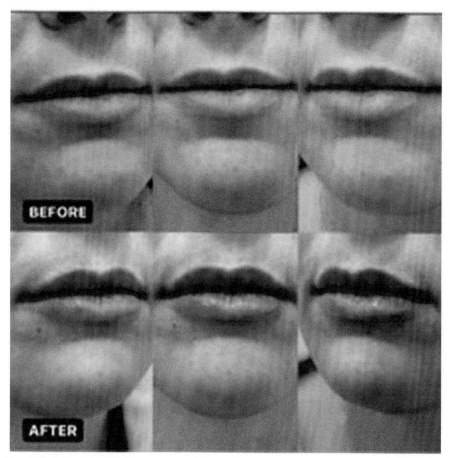

Fig. 2. Before and after: lip augmentation.

Kybella offers a minimally invasive, affordable alternative to a submental liposuction.[13,14] The effects of the treatment are likely to last a few years and may even possibly be permanent, particularly in the absence of significant weight gain. However, this has not yet been confirmed.[12] As with any procedure, however, there are risks that should be recognized. For Kybella treatments, risks include erythema, edema, pain, numbness, bruising, and induration at the treated areas. More serious effects include dysphagia and marginal mandibular nerve injury.[11]

Technique
At each Kybella treatment, the patient receives multiple small injections under the chin. The exact number of injections depends on the amount of fat under the chin and desired profiles. Each Kybella treatment session is given at least 1 month apart, with no more than 6 treatments in total.[15]

Concluding remarks
Seventy-nine percent of Kybella-treated patients reported high satisfaction with their face and chin appearance.[13] With its ability to permanently and effectively

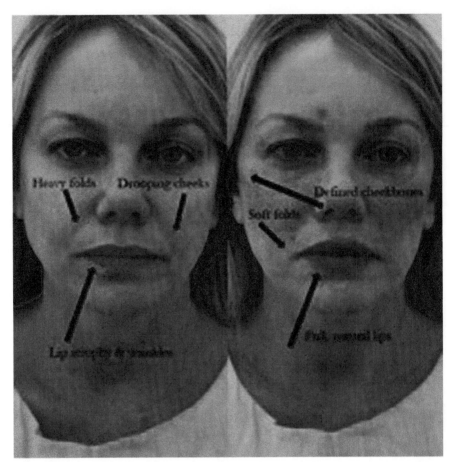

Fig. 3. Before and after: neurotoxin and fillers (cheekbones, undereyes, nasolabial folds, lips).

dissolve fat under the chin after multiple treatments, Kybella is a popular option for those looking for a noninvasive procedure rather than submental liposuction or a neck lift (**Fig. 12**).

SKIN RESURFACING

Resurfacing techniques treat skin surface irregularities, including actinic damage; pigmentation disorders; and changes caused by aging, such as wrinkling.[5] These techniques produce a controlled injury that must be the proper depth to treat the targeted pathology and achieve the desired result.[5]

Aging and actinic damage affect the epidermis and dermis. Aging causes epidermal hyperplasia, atrophy, and dysplasia, leading to an atrophic and flat epidermis. Dermal connective tissue shows progressive diminution with great loss of the reticular dermis. Over time, collagen fibers become degenerated and thick. Less collagen leads to thinning of the skin. Aging also causes loss of dermoepidermal papillae and melanocytes reduction. Actinically damaged skin exhibits elastosis, the presence of thickened, degraded elastic fibers.[5]

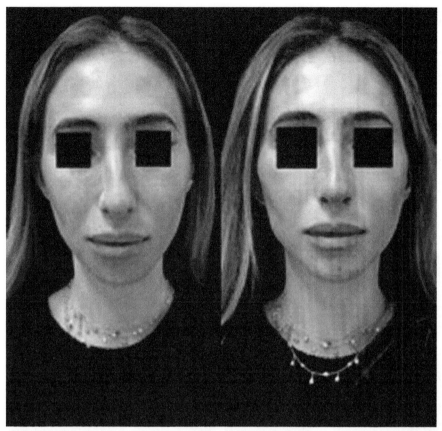

Fig. 4. Before and after: neurotoxin and fillers (cheekbones, undereyes, nose, lips, jawline, chin).

Individuals concerned about the surface of their skin, either regarding changes caused by aging, acne, or pigmentation differences, are good candidates for skin resurfacing procedures. The use of lasers, chemical peels, and microneedling can lead to the stimulation of new collagen and elastin, the removal of abnormal tissue, and an overall rejuvenation of the skin. Nevertheless, the use of these procedures is technique dependent, and numerous factors affect penetration and the depth of injury. Additionally, the risk of prolonged erythema or pigment loss is directly proportional to the depth of resurfacing, and prolonged healing times and scarring may occur.[5]

Lasers

Laser resurfacing is a good solution for freckles, melasma, age spots, and fine lines around the eyes and mouth. Laser treatment works well in combination with surgical procedures, such as a facelift or blepharoplasty. In 2016, more than 315,000 laser skin resurfacing procedures took place, making it the eighth most common nonsurgical procedure.[8]

Lasers send out high-energy light pulses, which are absorbed by water and chromophores, substances of the skin. The light from the laser transforms into heat energy, which then targets small sections of the skin, layer by layer.

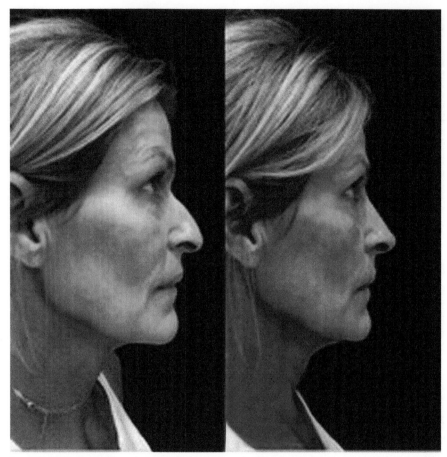

Fig. 5. Middle aged female patient before and after nonsurgical rhinoplasty. Notice a decrease in appearance of the dorsal hump and an uplifted tip creating a defined tip and sloped bridge.

During the healing process, new skin grows to replace the skin treated by the laser.[16]

The ablation depth of lasers is controlled precisely and thus lasers are characterized as either ablative or nonablative.[17] Ablative lasers vaporize the superficial layers of the skin by heating the dermis to stimulate new collagen production by fibroblasts.[1] Ablative lasers commonly use pulsed carbon dioxide and erbium:YAG laser wavelengths.[17] On average, carbon dioxide systems ablate 20 to 60 μm of tissue with the initial pass, and the residual thermal damage extends to a depth of 20 to 100 μm after multiple passes, making them more useful for deep ablations.[17] The erbium:YAG pulse laser systems vaporize 2 to 5 μm of tissue per pass and leave behind a 20- to 50-μm zone of residual thermal damage, making them the better option for finely tuned light to medium ablations.[17] These laser systems aim to produce a significant degree of improvement with less skin wounding to generate fibroplasia and granulation but with thin zones of thermal damage.[17]

Nonablative lasers instead stimulate collagen growth only by creating focal thermal injury within the dermis.[17] The Q-switched neodymium:yttrium-aluminum-garnet laser

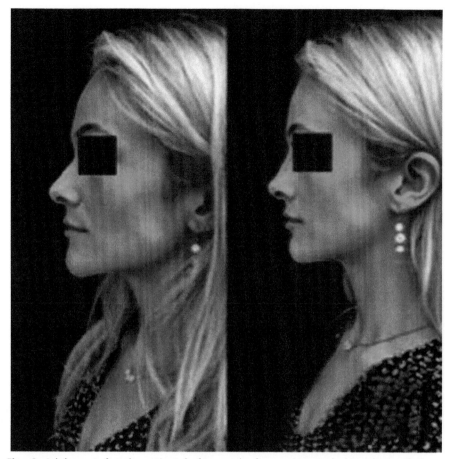

Fig. 6. Adolescent female patient before and after nonsurgical rhinoplasty. Notice a straightened dorsum and a lifted and defined tip.

is particularly useful in the treatment of periocular and perioral rhytides.[17] Other nonablative lasers include intense pulsed nonlaser light sources, diode lasers, and pulsed-dye lasers.[17] Fractional photothermolysis induces deep dermal damage that stimulates collagen synthesis and remodeling while producing minimal epidermal damage.[17] The laser procedures require only a short period of recovery time and the treated skin looks rejuvenated after 2 weeks. Treatment may require several sessions.[17]

Technique
The following standard set of techniques can be used as a protocol template. The face is first treated with three separate passes at 100 μm of ablation with no coagulation using a scanning pattern.[4] This produces a uniform depth of ablated tissue of 300 μm. The handpiece should be held a constant distance from the skin at a perpendicular angle.[4] After each pass, denuded skin is removed with sterile moist gauze and assessed for depth by noting the following clinical endpoints: wrinkle ablation, reticular punctate bleeding pattern, and lacey or fragmented appearance of midreticular dermis.[4] At the caudal border of the mandible, one should taper to

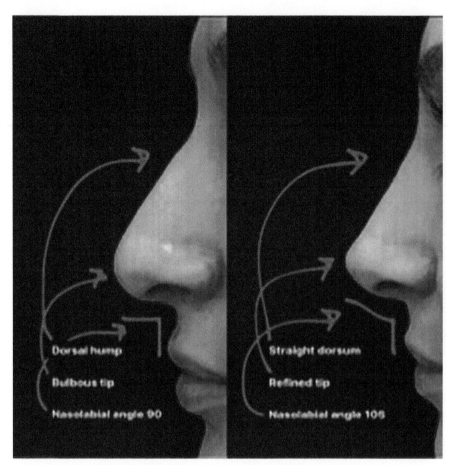

Fig. 7. Young female patient before and after nonsurgical rhinoplasty. Notice how microadjustments straightened the dorsum, defined the tip, and improved the nasolabial angle.

200 μm and then to 100 μm at the neck transition. Deeper rhytids should be spot treated with rapid fire 30 μm pulses.[4] To blend the laser-treated skin with the untreated skin, these transitional areas should be tapered by spot treating the margins using 30 μm of ablation. When skin tightening is needed, the surgeon can choose to add 25 μm of coagulation during the third pass, understanding that this could result in prolonged postoperative erythema.[4] Aquaphor is applied after the procedure to soothe the skin.

Concluding remarks

For a physician practicing laser resurfacing, an extensive knowledge of skin histology is required. Patients seeking significant improvement of their facial complexion should consider laser treatment, a principal noninvasive option.

Chemical Peels

Chemical peels are another option for skin resurfacing. Inexpensive, chemical peels are a generally safe treatment option for certain skin disorders and for refreshing the skin.[17] Specifically, chemical peels aim to improve fine lines, reduce sun spots,

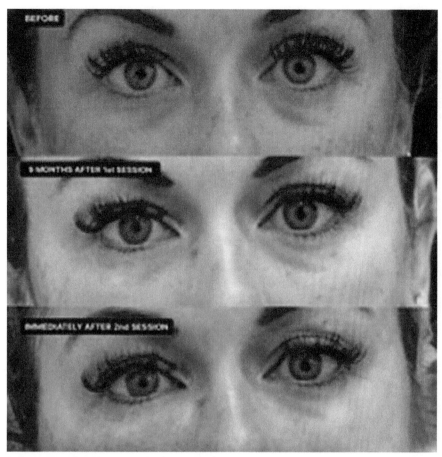

Fig. 8. Young female patient before and after two sessions of tear trough augmentation. Notice the improvement of her undereye hollows and darkness, and a softer more appealing lid-cheek junction.

and revitalize the complexion. In 2016, the chemical peel treatment was the fifth most common nonsurgical procedure in the United States, with more than 600,000 treatments taking place.[18]

Chemical peels are used to create an injury of a specified skin depth with the aim of stimulating new skin growth and improving surface appearance and texture.[18] The peels are classified by the depth of their action into the following categories: superficial, medium, and deep. Individual skin characteristics, healing time, and the area of skin to be treated should be considered for the most effective results.[18]

Superficial peels are useful in the treatment of acne, dyschromias, postinflammatory pigmentation, and in achieving skin radiance.[19] Medium-depth peels are used in the treatment of dyschromias, including solar lentigines, multiple keratosis, superficial scars, pigmentary disorders, and textural changes.[19] The healing process is longer than for a superficial peel, with full epithelialization occurring in approximately 1 week. Deep peels are often used for severe photoaging, deep or coarse wrinkles, scars, and occasionally precancerous skin lesions.[19] Deep peels, usually performed

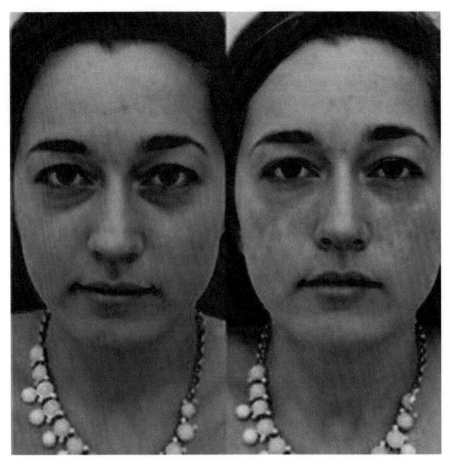

Fig. 9. Young female patient before and after tear trough augmentation. Notice an improvement in infraorbital hollows, dark circles, and puffiness under the eyes.

with phenol in combination with croton oil, cause rapid denaturization of surface keratin in the dermis and outer dermis.[19]

Technique

The application technique varies according to the peeling agent used. Liquid products may be applied with a brush, cotton tip applicator, or cotton or gauze swab. Gels are applied with a wooden spatula. The chemical peeling should start on areas of thicker skin. The forehead, cheeks, nose and chin are treated first, followed by the perioral and periorbital skin.[18] The peeling agent should be applied in an upward direction with firm even strokes and extended beyond the vermillion border and into the oral commissures. A feathering technique should be used at the edge of the treatment site to avoid sharp demarcation lines.[18] In areas of deep wrinkling, the physician should stretch the skin to prevent pooling of the peeling agent.[18]

Good post-procedure care ensures prompt recovery of the skin and prevents complications. A bland emollient should be applied regularly to the skin until peeling is complete. If crusting develops, a topical antibacterial agent may be prescribed. Makeup may be applied after re-epithelialization has taken place.

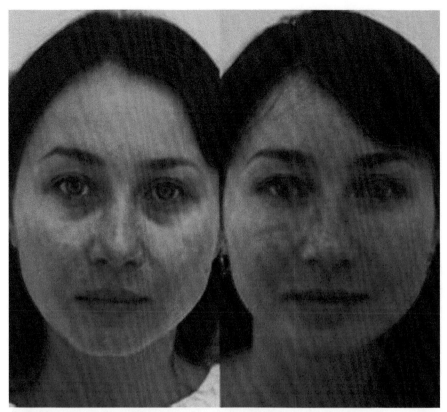

Fig. 10. Middle aged female patient before and after tear trough augmentation. Notice a softening in her lid-cheek junction and a smoother refreshed orbital hollow.

Although chemical peels are a safe procedure, adverse effects can occur following peeling and vary according to peel depth. Minor complications include irritation burning, erythema, pruritus, edema, and blistering.[18] Major complications, although rare, include allergic reactions, laryngeal edema, toxic shock syndrome, cardiotoxicity, salicylism, acute kidney injury, lower lid ectropion, corneal damage, significant scarring, and dyspigmentation.[18]

Concluding remarks

Chemical peels are a rapid, safe, and cost-effective technique for cutaneous rejuvenation. They are useful for specific dermatologic conditions, such as acne vulgaris, melisma, actinic karatoses, and scarring. Chemical peels are individualized to the patient's skincare needs.

Microneedling

Skin resurfacing continues with the rising popularity of the microneedling procedure. Microneedling is a therapy in which thin needles are rolled over the surface of the skin to induce rapidly healing micropunctures. The production of these microwounds initiates the postinflammatory chemical cascade and ultimately stimulates collagen production. Increased collagen production paired with elastin fiber production results in skin remodeling.[19] Microneedling is recommended to treat wrinkles caused by skin aging, scars, and stretch marks.[19,20]

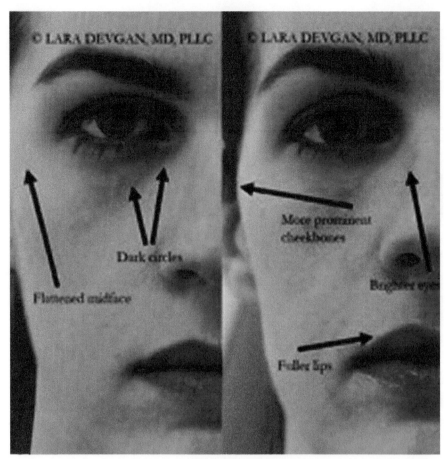

Fig. 11. Before and after: chin augmentation, lip augmentation, tear trough augmentation.

Many patients prefer microneedling to laser and chemical peels because it is safe for use in all skin tones, all parts of the body (including abdomen stretch marks), and all times of life (including pregnancy and breastfeeding). Because the epidermis is retained, microneedling comes with lower risk of infection, postinflammatory hyperpigmentation, and scarring compared with other resurfacing modalities.[18] In addition, the recovery time with microneedling is short, with mild redness usually lasting less than a day, as compared with 1 week or more with laser or peels.

Technique

Topical anesthesia with lidocaine and prilocaine cream (EMLA) is applied to the area to be treated and covered with cellophane tape for 15 to 45 minutes. The cream is then removed using normal saline. An antiseptic solution is then applied, right before the microneedling procedure begins.[19]

The skin of the face is stretched by one hand while the other hand is used to roll the instrument over in a direction perpendicular to that of stretching force. The roller is rolled 15 to 20 times in horizontal, vertical, and both oblique directions.[23] The base of the scar should be treated. Pinpoint bleeding should occur from the base of the scar. Saline pads are kept over the treated area.

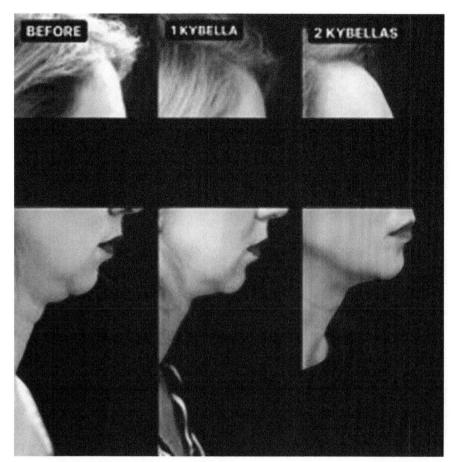

Fig. 12. Before and after: Kybella treatments.

The treated area is swollen and superficially bruised. It should be covered with damp swabs that are replaced every 2 hours to absorb the bleeding and serous discharge. Topical antibiotic cream is applied for a few days to minimize the chance of bacterial infection. Patients are told to avoid sun exposure and strong chemicals or any facial cosmetic procedure for at least 1 week.[23]

Complications for the procedure are almost negligible. Poor-quality needles of the roller device often lead to bending at needle tips after multiple treatments, which results in more tissue damage. Overaggressive needling using a tattoo gun may also cause scarring.[23]

Concluding remarks

Microneedling is an alternative for those reluctant to try neurotoxins or fillers but are concerned with their complexions. Improved skin appearance is evident almost immediately and continues for 4 to 6 weeks. In a previous microneedling study, patients reported an 80% to 85% overall satisfaction with the therapy.[20] Overall, the microneedling treatment is a painless skin resurfacing option with minimal chemical exposure and short recovery time (**Fig. 13**).

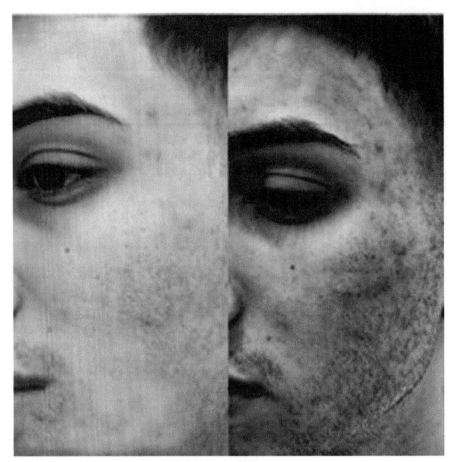

Fig. 13. Before and after: microneedling.

SUMMARY

Minimally invasive techniques to address facial irregularities, including injectables of neurotoxin, dermal fillers, and deoxycholic acid, and skin resurfacing peels, lasers, and microneedling, are less invasive alternatives and are part of a custom combination of procedures that achieves individually tailored results. Unlike surgery, these procedures serve as minimal-downtime treatments for fine lines, sun damage, irregular pigmentation, or textural issues. A thorough consultation between the practicing surgeon and patient can create a successful treatment plan to optimally address facial desires and concerns.

REFERENCES

1. Chuang J. Overview of facial plastic surgery and current developments. Surg J 2016. https://doi.org/10.1055/s-0036-1572360.
2. Sykes JM, Trevidic P, Suárez GA, et al. Newer understanding of specific anatomic targets in the aging face as applied to injectables. Plast Reconstr Surg 2015;136. https://doi.org/10.1097/prs.0000000000001731.

3. Funt D, Pavicic T. Dermal fillers in aesthetics. Plast Surg Nurs 2015;35(1):13–32.
4. Monheit G. Neurotoxins. Plast Reconstr Surg 2015;136. https://doi.org/10.1097/prs.0000000000001771.
5. Aston SJ, Rees TD. Aesthetic plastic surgery. Philadelphia: Saunders; 1980.
6. Wu DC, Fabi SG, Goldman MP. Neurotoxins. Plast Reconstr Surg 2015;136. https://doi.org/10.1097/prs.0000000000001750.
7. Chang BL, Wilson AJ, Taglienti AJ, et al. Patient perceived benefit in facial aesthetic procedures: FACE-Q as a tool to study botulinum toxin injection outcomes. Aesthet Surg J 2016;36(7):810–20.
8. American Society of Plastic Surgeons. Available at: https://www.plasticsurgery.org/reconstructive-procedures. Accessed June 12, 2018.
9. Hellings PW, Trenité GJN. Long-term patient satisfaction after revision rhinoplasty. Laryngoscope 2007;117(6):985–9.
10. Vedamurthy M, Vedamurthy A. Dermal fillers: tips to achieve successful outcomes. J Cutan Aesthet Surg 2008;1(2):64.
11. Carruthers J, Carruthers A, Humphrey S. Introduction to fillers. Plast Reconstr Surg 2015;136. https://doi.org/10.1097/prs.0000000000001770.
12. Shah GM, Greenberg JN, Tanzi EL, et al. Noninvasive approach to treatment of submental fullness. Semin Cutan Med Surg 2017;36(4):164–9.
13. Kirk D, Gart L, Ferneini E. Deoxycholic acid injection for the reduction of submental fat in adults. J Oral Maxillofac Surg 2016;74(9). https://doi.org/10.1016/j.joms.2016.06.091.
14. Cohen J. Additional thoughts on the new treatment Kybella. Semin Cutan Med Surg 2015;34(3):138–9.
15. Kybella. Kybella. Available at: https://www.mykybella.com/. Accessed June 18, 2018.
16. Alster T. Laser skin resurfacing. Cosmetic Dermatology 2005. https://doi.org/10.1007/3-540-27333-6_7.
17. Rendon MI. Evidence and considerations in the application of chemical peels in skin disorders and aesthetic resurfacing. J Clin Aesthet Dermatol 2010;3(7):32–43.
18. Hogan S. Microneedling: a new approach for treating textural abnormalities and scars. Semin Cutan Med Surg 2017. https://doi.org/10.12788/j.sder.2017.042.
19. Nair P. Microneedling. Treasure Island (FL): StatPearls Publishing; 2018.
20. Iriarte C, Awosika O, Rengifo-Pardo M, et al. Review of applications of microneedling in dermatology. Clin Cosmet Investig Dermatol 2017;10:289–98.

Mohs Reconstruction and Scar Revision

Andrew W. Joseph, MD, MPH[a],*, Shannon S. Joseph, MD[b]

KEYWORDS

- Facial plastic surgery • Head and neck reconstruction • Skin cancer • Mohs excision
- Scar revision

KEY POINTS

- Patients should be carefully selected when considering for office-based reconstruction following Mohs. Those patients with significant medical comorbidities, those with a history of significant anxiety, or those expected to require more extensive reconstructive procedures are better suited for repair in the operating room.
- Most office-based cutaneous defect reconstructions are accomplished with local flaps or skin grafting procedures.
- Scar management is an important aspect of successful facial reconstruction, and available techniques include surgical scar revision, scar irregularization, skin resurfacing, and adjunctive techniques.

INTRODUCTION

Over the past 20 years, Mohs micrographic surgery (MMS) has become a commonly used surgical option in treating certain cutaneous malignancies. Although defects following MMS can be extensive and require an operating room (OR) setting for reconstruction, office-based repairs are frequently possible. Approaches to facial reconstruction have been well described in many texts.[1–3] This article aims to discuss the clinical considerations and surgical techniques for office-based reconstruction of soft tissue defects and management of scars.

Considerations for Office-Based Reconstructive Procedures Following Mohs

Patient selection

The success of office-based reconstructions can be highly dependent on correct patient selection. All patients should ideally be evaluated by the reconstructive surgeon

Disclosure Statement: The authors have nothing to disclose.
[a] Facial Plastic and Reconstructive Surgery, Department of Otolaryngology–Head and Neck Surgery, University of Michigan Medical School, 1904 Taubman Center, Ann Arbor, MI 48109, USA; [b] Department of Ophthalmology and Visual Sciences, University of Michigan Medical School, 714 Kellogg Eye Center, Ann Arbor, MI 48109, USA
* Corresponding author.
E-mail address: josephan@umich.edu

before the ablative procedure. This consultation is imperative because it allows the reconstructive surgeon to assess patients' history and determine whether they will be good candidates for office-based reconstruction.

Past medical, surgical, and social history should be thoroughly elicited during a consultation. Surgeons should specifically inquire about a history of prior head and neck surgical or radiation procedures, history of scleroderma or Ehlers-Danlos syndrome, and recent or active tobacco use. Furthermore, all patients should be explicitly asked about prior cardiac, pulmonary, or hematologic history. Patients with significant medical comorbidities (eg, significant cardiac dysfunction, poor pulmonary reserve or requiring home oxygen, history of bleeding diathesis) are better suited for reconstruction in the OR setting. The American Society of Anesthesiologists (ASA) classification can be used for risk stratification of patients.[4] Patients who are categorized as ASA I or II are suitable candidates for reconstructions in an office-based setting.

Another important aspect of the history to obtain is whether patients have anxiety or other psychiatric disorders, or other conditions preventing them from being able to remain stationary in a reclined position for the duration of the procedure. These patients are better suited for reconstruction in the OR under sedation.

Last, although data do not suggest that the duration of an office-based procedure is associated with increased risk of complications, the authors limit their procedures to those expected to take less than 2 to 3 hours.[5]

Surgical equipment and supplies

The reconstruction of most MMS defects requires only basic surgical instruments, a monopolar or bipolar cautery, and an overhead procedure room light. The instruments the authors use are listed in **Box 1**. It is also helpful to have a medical assistant or nurse who is familiar with sterile OR techniques available during the procedure.

Box 1
Suggested common surgical instruments for minor office-based reconstructive procedures

Suggested minor procedure instrument set

1. Small Iris scissors straight
2. Small Iris scissors curved
3. Small Stevens tenotomy scissors curved
4. Gorney facelift scissors
5. Small suture scissors
6. Brown forceps (2)
7. Adson forceps (2)
8. Iris tissue forceps or Castroviejo suturing forceps 0.5 mm (2)
9. Mosquito hemostat straight (2)
10. Mosquito hemostat curved (2)
11. Needle holder (2)
12. Scalpel handle
13. Towel clips (2)

Number in bracket denotes quantity of an instrument

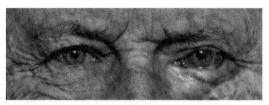

Fig. 1. Cicatricial ectropion of left lower eyelid resulting from vertical shortening of the anterior lamella.

APPROACHES TO CUTANEOUS RECONSTRUCTION
Principles in Facial Reconstruction

When planning a reconstruction, the authors find it helpful to consider several factors, as follows: (1) borders of aesthetic regions, (2) relaxed skin tension lines (RSTLs), (3) areas of available tissue recruitment, and (4) immobile structures or landmarks that should remain undistorted. Together these factors guide the selection of reconstructive techniques.

Facial aesthetic regions

The face has a complex 3-dimensional anatomy and may be conceptualized as a network of valleys and peaks that form natural facial aesthetic regions (FAR). A keen understanding of these regions is essential for successful reconstruction. The major FARs consist of the forehead, periocular areas, cheeks, lips, chin, nose, and auricles. These regions may be further divided into smaller subunits.[1,3] In addition to the contour differences among the FARs, there are also notable variations in skin thickness and sebaceous gland density across the regions.

Relaxed skin tension lines

For scars of facial reconstruction to be as inconspicuous as possible, they should be positioned in areas where they are maximally camouflaged. In the head and neck region, these areas include hair-bearing skin (scalp), within the nose or mouth, within the postauricular area, or in the submental region. In situations where this is not possible, scars are best placed along borders between FARs or parallel to RSTLs.

Soft tissue recruitment

When planning facial reconstruction, it is helpful to identify areas where ample soft tissue may be recruited within a given FAR. The regions vary tremendously in skin extensibility and the amount of redundant tissue available for recruitment. The cheek is generally the most forgiving region, with a large amount of tissue available for recruitment along the medial and buccal cheek regions, and, to lesser extent, along the lateral cheek. The nasal skin envelope has a relatively small amount of tissue available for recruitment, whereas the forehead often allows for a moderate amount tissue recruitment. The lips have a limited amount of cutaneous tissue, so local flaps in this region often require the recruitment of tissue from the relatively mobile adjacent medial cheek.

Immobile structures

The face has certain immobile structures and landmarks that should not be disturbed during reconstruction. Otherwise, unfavorable functional and aesthetic outcomes may result. Within the upper face, the anterior hairline, temporal hair tufts, and brows should be maintained in their native position. Within the midface, it is critical to avoid any amount of tension on the lower eyelids and/or lateral canthal area, especially in older patients. Vertical tension on these anatomic structures can result in eyelid ectropion, retraction, and subsequent exposure keratopathy (**Fig. 1**). Within the lateral cheek, the lobule position can be easily distorted. Closure adjacent to the lobule should not be under tension, as a pixie ear deformity may result. Last, the alar margin is an easily disturbed landmark, where even 1-mm deviations can result in unsightly amounts of alar retraction.

Reconstructive Techniques

There are many surgical techniques in the armamentarium of the facial reconstructive surgeon. The reconstructive ladder can help surgeons conceptualize these techniques in a systematic manner (**Fig. 2**). Within the office setting, reconstruction most commonly involves primary closure, local flaps, and skin grafts. In certain situations, interpolated flaps may also be performed in an office setting, although the authors prefer to perform these under anesthesia because they generally require more extensive dissection and can result in bleeding into/around the eyes.

Patient preparation

Beyond appropriate patient selection and judicious surgical planning, one of the most important aspects of performing successful in-office reconstructive procedures is patient preparation. Given that procedures are performed while the patient is awake, much attention should be directed to making the procedure area as comfortable as possible for the patient as well as for the surgeon. The procedure room should be equipped with an adjustable table or procedure chair (**Fig. 3**). The patient is generally situated supine with a ring-style cushion, which provides the patient with comfort without being obstructive for the surgeon. If the patient is agreeable, it is often helpful to provide relaxing background music. Preprocedure oral anxiolytics are helpful for select patients with history of anxiety, although the patients would then require a driver to and from the procedure.

After positioning of the patient, the surgical area is injected with a local anesthetic. The authors use a combination of 1% lidocaine with 1:100,000 epinephrine mixed equally with 0.25% bupivacaine, because this provides both a rapid onset of action and a prolonged anesthetic effect. In patients who are highly averse to needles, various topical anesthetic preparations or ice may be used before the introduction of needles.

Reconstruction of forehead defects

Small (<2 cm) and some medium-sized (<3 cm) forehead defects may be suitable for reconstruction in the office. Within the forehead, bilateral supraorbital and supratrochlear nerve blocks can provide substantial anesthesia and can be performed before wider administration of local anesthetic to the rest of the forehead.

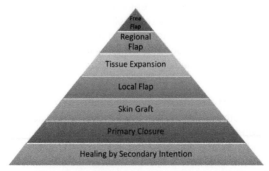

Fig. 2. Wound management options of varying complexity are illustrated by the reconstructive ladder.

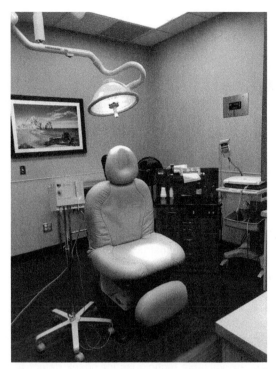

Fig. 3. Typical procedure room with procedure chair, cautery, and overhead lighting.

For most of the forehead, RSTLs are situated horizontally, and scars are often placed parallel to or within rhytids. The exception to this rule pertains to the midline portion of the forehead, where the galeal midline raphe exists and vertical closures are often acceptable.

Undermining in the forehead is generally accomplished easily within the subgaleal plane, which is avascular. Although undermining within the subcutaneous plane may result in greater skin recruitment per undermined surface area, it may be associated with more forehead hypesthesia postoperatively.

Local advancement flaps are the most common techniques used to close forehead defects. Small and medium-sized defects of the midline or paramedian forehead may be closed vertically or horizontally; the decision is based on the orientation of the long axis of the defect. Defects with the long axis situated horizontally may be closed by advancement of tissue superior and/or inferior to the defect, so long as the brow position is not adversely impacted (**Fig. 4**). The ideal position of the brows is at the level of the superior orbital rim in men, and just above the superior orbital rim in women. In older individuals with significant skin laxity, brow elevation of up to 1 cm may resolve spontaneously postoperatively due to gravity, although caution should be exercised in younger patients. Lateral forehead defects adjacent to the eyebrow may be closed with unilateral or bilateral advancement flaps in an "H-plasty" configuration (**Fig. 5**). Alternatively, in patients without well-defined horizontal rhytids within which the scars of an H-plasty could be camouflaged, "A-to-T" closures are a good option for reconstruction. Various rotation-advancement flaps may also be used for lateral forehead reconstruction.

For large forehead defects where complete closure is expected to be difficult, the defect could first be significantly reduced in size with advancement flaps. The

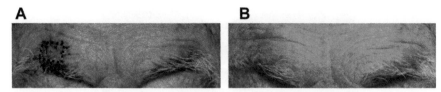

Fig. 4. Horizontal advancement closure of lateral forehead defect. (*A*) Preoperative photograph with melanoma square emphasized by stippled marking. (*B*) Three-month postoperative result.

remaining open defect can then be left to heal by secondary intention. Compared with skin grafting, healing by secondary intention can often result in more acceptable results and may be serially excised later.

Reconstruction of cheek defects

Cheek defects are well suited for reconstruction in the office setting because it is well tolerated under local anesthetic.

Most cheek defects are closed with local flaps. Undermining is carried out in the subcutaneous plane for a distance up to 3 to 4 cm, beyond which little additional recruitment will result. Primary repair or closure with bilateral advancement flaps is often a good choice for defects adjacent to FAR borders (eg, melolabial crease). In cases where the scar cannot be placed within an FAR border, an attempt is made to place the scar parallel to the RSTLs.

Transposition flaps are valuable techniques for cheek defect reconstruction. The choice of which transposition flap to use depends on defect size, location, and shape. The note flap, rhombic flap, and Z-plasty are all commonly used. If a rhombic flap is chosen, the authors find the Dufourmentel modification to be versatile and useful.[6] This modification is created by extending a line from the short axis of the flap, and a second line parallel to one of the sides of the defect. The angle created from these 2 lines is bisected with a line equal in length to the side of the rhomboid, and this forms the first side of the flap. The second side of the flap is then formed by extension of a line parallel to the long axis of the parallelogram (**Fig. 6**). Regardless of the exact flap used, the surgeon should always attempt to achieve recruitment in a lateral or medial direction and minimize vertical tension on the lower eyelid.

The "V-to-Y" subcutaneous pedicled island advancement flap is a good technique for reconstruction of medial cheek defects that abut the melolabial crease or nasal base. For this flap, a triangular island of skin is outlined inferior to the defect. The width

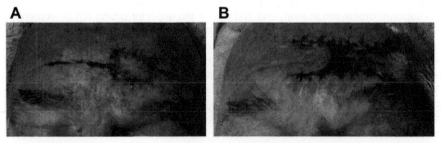

Fig. 5. H-plasty closure of left forehead defect. (*A*) Preoperative defect with melanoma square outlined with sutures. (*B*) Intraoperative photograph immediately following repair.

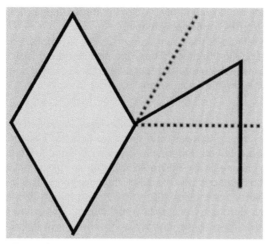

Fig. 6. Dufourmentel modification of the rhombic flap.

of this island is usually equal to the width of the defect, and the apex of the triangle is positioned within the melolabial fold. Skin incisions are made around the island of skin and taken into the subcutaneous level. Incisions into the subcutaneous fat may be beveled outward to help preserve as much of a subcutaneous pedicle as possible, and the surgeon should ensure that dissection remains superficial to the facial mimetic muscles.

Larger defects of the medial cheek may be closed with a variety of rotational-advancement flaps; defects requiring cervicofacial flaps are better performed under general anesthetic.

Reconstruction of lip defects

Lips defect reconstruction can be challenging under local anesthetic, and patients should be selected carefully based on size of the defect and affected aesthetic sub-units. Defects that are greater than one-third of the horizontal width of the lip are likely better reconstructed under sedation or general anesthetic. Before injection of local anesthetic, it is important to mark the precise location of the vermillion border. For lower lip reconstruction, it is helpful to place 4 × 4 gauze in the gingivolabial and/or gingivobuccal sulcus to collect blood that could drain into the mouth. Digital pressure on the lip is usually more than adequate to limit bleeding, but one must be prepared to ligate the superior or inferior labial artery if needed. Small cutaneous-only defects can be closed in a primary fashion, with the incision oriented radially, parallel to the RSTLs. In patients with limited tissue for advancement closure, the defect may be converted to full thickness and then closed in 3 layers (oral mucosa, orbicularis oris muscle, and skin) in a wedge configuration.

Reconstruction of nasal defects

Select nasal cutaneous defects may be reconstructed in the office under local anesthesia. It should be noted that although aggressive histology, recurrent lesions, and significant ulceration are suggestive of more extensive involvement, it is often difficult to predict which nasal lesions will result in significant post-Mohs defects requiring the OR for optimal reconstruction. Cutaneous malignancies involving subunits, such as the nasal ala, columella, and soft triangle, may be better suited for repair in the OR because these areas more commonly require intranasal flaps or additional grafts that are more easily performed under anesthesia.

Small (<1.5 cm) defects of the nasal dorsum, nasal sidewalls, and nasal tip are the most suitable for repair in the office. There are a multitude of factors that impact the choice of reconstructive techniques for nasal defects. The most commonly used techniques will be outlined in later discussion.

Nasal bilobe flap

The nasal bilobe flap is one of the most common local flaps used for reconstruction of small nasal dorsum, nasal sidewall, and nasal tip defects. Because the entire nasal soft tissue envelope requires undermining, the reconstruction should be preceded by 8 to 10 mL of local anesthetic infiltrated into the soft tissue envelope of the entire nose. Modern reconstructions use the Zitelli modification to the bilobe flap because it results in a smaller arc of rotation (90° vs 180° with the traditional flap), a reduced standing cutaneous deformity, and less trapdooring.[7] The base of the bilobe flap can be situated either medially or laterally and depends on the size and location of the defect. When possible, the flap is designed so that the linear scar that forms after closure of the secondary lobe donor site is situated at the junction of the dorsum-sidewall aesthetic subunit boundary. The primary and secondary lobes are then drawn on the skin using a precise geometric technique to ensure consistent results.[2] The nasal bilobe flap commonly requires dermabrasion, which may be performed as early as 6 weeks postoperatively.

Note flap

Similar to the nasal bilobe flap, the note flap is a transposition flap that is very useful for small cutaneous nasal defects involving less-thick skin.[8] This flap takes a configuration that is similar to a musical eighth note and is designed by drawing a tangent to the cutaneous defect that is approximately 1.5 times the diameter of the defect (**Fig. 7**). A second line is extended from the end of the tangent line at an angle of approximately 50° to –60°, thus forming a triangular-shaped flap. Wide undermining takes place in the subfascial plane, and the triangular flap is transposed into position. The standing cutaneous deformity is excised at the base of the defect before skin closure.

Full-thickness skin graft

Full-thickness skin grafts are frequently used for defects involving the nasal tip, dorsum, and nasal sidewall. Patients with Fitzpatrick 1 or 2 skin type and less sebaceous skin are the best candidates for skin grafting. Skin grafts are commonly harvested from the supraclavicular or postauricular areas and then thinned to an appropriate thickness. The nasal tip, sidewalls, and caudal aspect of the dorsum are relatively thicker and require less thinning of the graft. The graft is fashioned to match the size of the defect or slightly larger. A bolster dressing is fixated into position over the graft for 5 to 7 days after the procedure.

SCAR MANAGEMENT

To obtain the best possible reconstructive results, significant attention should be paid to postoperative management of scars. This section offers practical recommendations for evaluation and management of facial scars.

Evaluation of Facial Scars

A multitude of factors can contribute to the development of aesthetically unappealing scars. Almost all incisions have a conspicuous appearance during the first month after

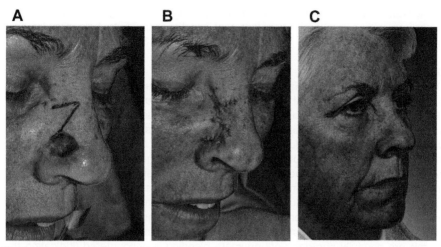

Fig. 7. Note flap for repair of sidewall defect. (*A*) Design of note flap. (*B*) Completed closure of defect. (*C*) One-year postoperative result. (*From* Joseph AW, Truesdale C, Baker SR. Reconstruction of the nose. Facial Plast Surg Clin 2019;27(1):47. Originally Figure 4; with permission.)

a procedure, due to the inflammatory and early proliferative phases of wound healing. Scars then slowly improve in appearance during the maturation phase, which extends from approximately 3 weeks to up to 1 year after a procedure. In the early postoperative period, patients require reassurance that scars will continue to improve in appearance and often do not require any further treatment.

Scar evaluation should begin with a thorough history, including the date of surgical procedure, history of hypertrophic scars or keloids, history of sun exposure, and examination of other traumatic or surgical scars. Evaluation of the scar in question should focus on the following 5 attributes: (1) location, (2) orientation, (3) color/vascularity, (4) width, and (5) texture/depth. Scar location may be described by its position within the FARs. Orientation of scars should be considered with regard to RSTLs as well as the boundaries of adjacent FARs. Scar color can vary depending on time from surgery/injury as well as ethnic background, but can be described with regard to adjacent uninvolved skin (eg, pink, hyperpigmented, hypopigmented). In addition, scars may develop vascular hyperplasia, which should be documented. An ideal scar should be no wider than 1 mm. Widened scars may develop for a variety of reasons, the most common of which is excessive skin tension during wound closure. Finally, skin texture and depth (or elevation) of a scar should be noted.

Management of Facial Scars

Comprehensive management of scars is outside the scope of this article; this section discusses common scar management modalities that can be used in the office setting.

Conservative management

There are a variety of nonsurgical scar management techniques. Following a procedure, after epithelialization is complete, the authors recommend usage of silicone sheets (generally left in place for at least 12 hours) or twice a day silicone gel application. The exact mechanism of silicone has not been elucidated, but it may help to preserve or improve scar hydration.[9] The authors generally recommend continuation of these treatments for 6 to 12 months. They also recommend regular application of a sunscreen with a sun protection factor of greater than 35 to help prevent scar hyperpigmentation.

Dermabrasion

Dermabrasion is an essential technique that softens scars with irregular texture through mechanical removal of the epidermis and superficial dermis. It should be noted that laser skin resurfacing with a CO_2 or Er:YAG laser is an excellent alternative to dermabrasion, but not all practices have this resource at their disposal. Contraindications to dermabrasion include history of scleroderma, active bacterial or viral skin infections, or use of isotretinoin within the past year. Dermabrasion may be performed with either a high-speed powered diamond or wire brush fraise. Smaller scars may be treated with sterilized medium-grit sandpaper. Dermabrasion is commonly performed in the office, but this procedure can result in significant aerosolization of skin debris and blood. As such, appropriate personal protective equipment should be donned at all times. After the administration of local anesthetic, the epidermis and superficial dermis are carefully abraded until punctate bleeding is encountered (indicating the papillary dermis has been entered). Petroleum is applied several times a day to the dermabraded areas until full epithelialization has occurred (usually within a week).

Surgical excision

Some scars that are widened, irregular, or hypertrophic may need surgical revision. Traumatic scars have a higher likelihood of requiring surgical revision, and it is advantageous to counsel these patients after the initial repair that secondary procedures may be necessary. The key to achieving good outcomes following surgical scar revisions is a meticulous, tension-free closure. When performing scar revisions on the cheek or forehead, the epidermis is excised sharply in a fusiform pattern, while preserving deep dermis and/or underlying scar tissue. Preservation of this deeper scar tissue allows for a platform on which the revised closure can rest and helps to prevent depression of the scar. Closure is achieved in a layered fashion. With scar revisions, the authors often seek to achieve good eversion of wound edges with a combination of vertical mattress and simple interrupted skin sutures (the authors generally use a 5-0 or 6-0 monofilament nonabsorbable suture to approximate the skin edges). Sutures are removed 5 to 7 days following a scar revision.

Scar irregularization

Even the thinnest scars may be conspicuous and unsightly if they are lengthy, do not follow RSTLs, or are not situated at the borders of FARs. These scars are good candidates for techniques of irregularization, which relies on the principle that attention is drawn less to irregular lines as compared with linear lines. The main techniques for irregularization include geometric broken line pattern (GBLP), W-plasty, and Z-plasty. GBLP creates the most irregular line through the use of a random pattern of geometric-shaped flaps (eg, square, triangle, half circle) with complementary patterns drawn on the opposite side of the scar (**Fig. 8**). Each pattern should be ideally approximately 6 mm, and no more than 8 mm in width.

Adjunctive scar treatments

Other nonsurgical modalities can be used in scar management. Scar hyperpigmentation is often managed conservatively with observation or with topical bleaching creams, such as hydroquinone. Hydroquinone is available in a variety of formulations but is generally applied twice a day for 2 to 3 months.

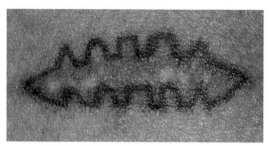

Fig. 8. Linear scar marked for GBLP irregularization.

Prolonged erythema and vascular hyperproliferation occasionally develop around scars. In these situations, broadband light treatment or pulsed-dye laser may be used in a series of 2 to 3 treatments to improve the appearance.

SUMMARY

Many facial cutaneous defects may be safely reconstructed in the office setting. Meticulous patient selection and preparation are critical. Local flaps and skin grafts are used for most office-based reconstructions, although additional techniques are possible. There are a variety of scar management modalities available to optimize the final reconstructive outcome.

REFERENCES

1. Baker SR. Local flaps in facial reconstruction. Philadelphia: Elsevier/Saunders; 2014. Available at: https://www.clinicalkey.com/dura/browse/bookChapter/3-s2.0-C20120004012. Accessed February 5, 2018.
2. Baker SR. Principles of nasal reconstruction. New York: Springer Science+Business Media, LLC; 2011. SpringerLink (Online service). Available at: https://doi.org/10.1007/978-0-387-89028-9. Accessed February 5, 2018.
3. Sherris D, Larrabee WF. Principles of facial reconstruction: a subunit approach to cutaneous repair. 2nd edition. New York: Thieme; 2009.
4. Quraishi SA. Anesthesia and analgesia for facial cosmetic procedures. In: Fedok FG, Carniol PJ, editors. Minimally invasive and office-based procedures in facial plastic surgery. SStuttgart, Germany: Thieme; 20.
5. Phillips BT, Wang ED, Rodman AJ, et al. Anesthesia duration as a marker for surgical complications in office-based plastic surgery. Ann Plast Surg 2012;69(4): 408–11.
6. Clark JM, Wang TD. Local flaps in scar revision. Facial Plast Surg 2001;17(4): 295–308.
7. Zitelli JA. The bilobed flap for nasal reconstruction. Arch Dermatol 1989;125(7): 957.
8. Walike JW, Larrabee WF. The "Note Flap". Arch Otolaryngol 1985;111(7):430–3.
9. Monstrey S, Middelkoop E, Vranckx JJ, et al. Updated scar management practical guidelines: non-invasive and invasive measures. J Plast Reconstr Aesthet Surg 2014;67(8):1017–25.

Office-Based Sinus Surgery

Alok T. Saini, MD[a], Martin J. Citardi, MD[b], William C. Yao, MD[b],
Amber U. Luong, MD, PhD[b],*

KEYWORDS

- Office-based surgery • Balloon catheter dilation • Sinus surgery
- Steroid-eluting implant • Cryotherapy

KEY POINTS

- Patient selection is a critical element of successful office-based sinonasal procedures.
- It is essential to select patients with pathology that can be sufficiently addressed in the office.
- A variety of procedures, including balloon catheter dilation, traditional endoscopic sinus surgery, polypectomy, endoscopic placement of drug delivering sinus implants, and cryotherapy treatments are available to otolaryngologists in the office setting.
- A sufficient anesthetic routine with or without sedation improves patient tolerance of office-based sinonasal procedures.
- Treatment goals, outcomes, and complications are similar for office-based procedures when compared with procedures performed in the operating room.

 Video content accompanies this article at http://www.oto.theclinics.com.

INTRODUCTION

In the last decade, the frequency of office-based rhinologic surgery has risen dramatically. The development of balloon catheter dilation (BCD) has facilitated a transition of rhinologic procedures to the office setting. In addition, the development of novel technologies has expanded the boundaries of in-office surgery. A shift to lower-cost venues for health care delivery has also driven this shift in site of service for rhinology

Disclosure Statement: Dr A.U. Luong is a consultant to 480 Biomedical, Aerin Medical, ENTvantage, and Medtronic. She is on the speaker's bureau for Intersect ENT and Stryker. Dr M.J. Citardi serves as a consultant for Acclarent, Arrinex, Biosense Webster, Factory CRO, Intersect ENT, Medical Metrics, Medtronic, and Stryker. Drs W.C. Yao and A.U. Luong are Assistant and Associate Professors at the McGovern Medical School Department of Otorhinolaryngology, which receives industry research funding from Genetech and AstraZeneca.
[a] Department of Otorhinolaryngology–Head and Neck Surgery, University of Kentucky College of Medicine, 740 S. Limestone, E300E, Lexington, KY 40536, USA; [b] Department of Otorhinolaryngology–Head and Neck Surgery, McGovern Medical School, The University of Texas Health Science Center at Houston, Houston, TX, USA
* Corresponding author. 6431 Fannin Street, MSB 5.036, Houston, TX 77030.
E-mail address: amber.u.luong@uth.tmc.edu

Otolaryngol Clin N Am 52 (2019) 473–483
https://doi.org/10.1016/j.otc.2019.02.003
0030-6665/19/© 2019 Elsevier Inc. All rights reserved.

Abbreviations	
BCD	Balloon catheter dilation
CNS	Central nervous system
CRS	Chronic rhinosinusitis
CRSsNP	Chronic rhinosinusitis without polyposis
ESS	Endoscopic sinus surgery
RARS	Recurrent acute rhinosinusitis

procedures. In addition to BCD, cryotherapy of posterior nasal tissue, placement of drug-delivery sinus implants, polypectomies, and even traditional sinus surgery are performed routinely in the office-setting. A solid understanding of appropriate patient selection, appropriate surgical objectives, and available technology is critical to the implementation of successful office-based rhinology.

This article highlights the issues associated with some of the more common office-based sinus procedures, and provides practical information on set-up and reimbursement.

ROOM SET-UP, INSTRUMENTATION, AND SUPPLIES

A large initial investment to obtain the space, equipment, and supplies may be necessary to perform office-based sinonasal surgery successfully. The use of a procedure room may help the surgeon and the patient distinguish an office-based procedure from a routine clinic visit. Additionally, a designated procedure room can be structured in a manner that allows for optimal patient comfort while providing the surgeon with easy access to instruments and equipment to safely and effectively perform office-based surgery.

Before committing to performing in-office procedures, the surgeon must have appropriate staffing in place. The clinical staff must be trained in the care and usage of the equipment, which differs from that used during diagnostic office procedures. Because the patient is awake, it is important that the clinical staff work closely with the surgeon to ensure the appearance of an integrated and orchestrated workflow throughout the entire procedure. Importantly, billing staff must be coached so that they can optimize collections for these procedures.

The necessary equipment varies according to the planned procedure. At a minimum, each of these procedures requires a comfortable examination chair, a variety of nasal telescopes, a video tower, a camera, and a strong suction apparatus. A bright headlight is also a prerequisite. A full complement of endoscopic sinus surgical instruments is needed if traditional procedures are to be performed. These instruments must have a low profile for these procedures; in general, instruments with a pediatric designation are preferred even in the adult patient. Both through-cutting and grasping forceps are necessary. For frontal sinus work, giraffe forceps and frontal curettes are required. In general, not all instruments are used for all in-office cases, and thus, surgeons should instruct their staff about their anticipated instrument needs. Of course, all instruments should be easily available, because it is not possible to predict perfectly the course of each procedure.

Recently, navigation systems have been introduced for in-office use. The rationale for their application in an office setting is similar to the rationale during the early days of the introduction of navigation in the operating room. At that time, surgeons embraced this technology because they concluded that it allowed a more complete and thorough procedure. In the office setting, navigation can serve a similar function. In the awake patient, the addition of navigation may allow a more efficient completion of the surgical procedure.

Initially, navigation systems designed for the operating room setting were simply moved to an office location, but this approach is not optimal because of the unique constraints of the office setting. First, the available space in the office is much smaller; thus, all navigations intended for the office setting are much smaller than comparable systems designed for the operating room. For instance, Fiagon Navigation (Fiagon, Austin, TX) is a device that fits on a single shelf in the video cart, and Fusion Compact (Medtronic, Jacksonville, FL) places all functions in an all-in-one PC-monitor combination that contains the computer and screen. Set-up of the tracking system in an office setting has other special challenges. Both Fiagon and Fusion Compact attach their electromagnetic field generators directly to the patient chair. Precise placement is critical to avoid distortion (and even disruption) of the electromagnetic field. TruDi (Acclarent, Irvine, CA) has a unique arrangement of its field generator in a head and back rest that can block unwanted electromagnetic field interference from the metal in the examination chair.

Powered instrumentation (soft tissue shavers) has also been adapted for in-office use. These devices offer the advantage of a consistently sharp cutting blade and some systems are compatible with surgical navigation. Powered instrumentation also adds complexity and costs. Because they are noisy, patient acceptance may also be an issue.

Office procedures also require disposable supplies. For balloon sinus dilatation, the surgeon needs expensive sinus balloon kits available. If powered instrumentation is part of the plan, then a small variety of instrument tips must be purchased. Steroid-eluting sinus implants or middle meatal spacers may also need to be stocked in the clinic, if the surgeon includes these in his/her armamentarium. Finally, epistaxis supplies must be available for the management of bleeding. These supplies were originally intended for an operating room environment, and thus are more expensive than other ENT office supplies. Thus, the ENT office that begins to stock these materials must set up additional measures for inventory and financial controls.

Correct patient positioning is fundamental to the comfort of the surgeon and the patient. Many office procedure chairs offer additional padding for patient comfort and additional positional options. The procedure room set-up often mimics the operating room (**Figs. 1** and **2**) with the endoscopic and navigation screens directly in front of the

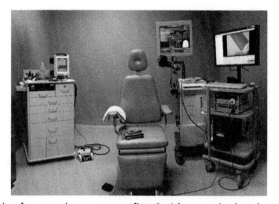

Fig. 1. An example of a procedure room outfitted with a standard otolaryngology workstation and an in-office navigation system and video tower.

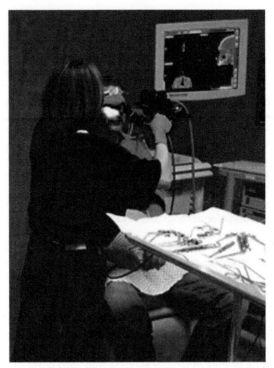

Fig. 2. During the procedure, the right-handed surgeon stands to the right of the patient, which is directly across from the navigation system and video tower.

surgeon and instruments nearby. Similarly, the operating surgeon may elect to have an assistant available to pass instruments in a scenario that is similar to the operating room. The patient is typically reclined to a comfortable position in the examination chair. The degree of recline is based on minimizing the degree of postnasal drainage of blood or secretions. Shorter surgeons may find it preferable to recline the patient, whereas this is less of an issue with taller surgeons.

PATIENT SELECTION AND EXPECTATIONS

Patient selection is a critical element of successful office-based sinonasal surgery. An overly anxious or sensitive patient undergoing an awake procedure in the clinic is almost certain to have a suboptimal outcome. Additionally, patients selected for office-based procedures must demonstrate pathology that can sufficiently be addressed in the clinic. These are the two most important factors in deciding when to pursue in-office surgery.

Certain patients are not amenable to awake procedures. An honest discussion with the patient is often all that is needed to make this determination. Patients tend to have good insight into their ability to tolerate an awake procedure. Many patients simply prefer to have procedures performed under general anesthesia. Others, however, may be willing to tolerate substantial interventions to avoid a formal operation. Allowing patients to guide such decisions is often adequate to successfully select patients for an office procedure.

A simple method of objectively determining one's suitability for an office-based surgery is assessing the patient's ability to tolerate rigid nasal endoscopy. A patient who tolerates endoscopy with interventions, such as debridement, is likely to tolerate a more extensive procedure. However, patients who are unable to cooperate in such situations are poor candidates, and it is wise to avoid pursuing in-office surgery in this circumstance.

One must always consider the comorbidities of the patient when selecting patients for office-based surgery. Patients on anticoagulation, generally, are considered poor candidates for in-office procedures. However, patients with significant comorbidities that make them high risk for undergoing general anesthesia may be candidates for in-office procedures requiring only local anesthesia.

Just as it is important to select patients capable of tolerating an awake procedure, it is essential to select patients with pathology that can be sufficiently addressed in the office. With technological advancements in recent years, an increasing variety and complexity of sinonasal diseases are being addressed in the office setting. Such diagnoses as sinus ostia stenosis, recurrent acute rhinosinusitis (RARS), or mild chronic rhinosinusitis without nasal polyps (CRSsNP) are commonly addressed with BCD. Management of recurrent nasal polyps in the office now has several procedure treatment options including polypectomies[1] and placement of steroid-eluting implants.[2] In addition, cryotherapy is offered for treatment of chronic rhinitis.[3] The complexity and variety of conditions treated in the office varies the most with traditional endoscopic sinus surgery (ESS). Biopsies of sinonasal tumors, management of maxillary sinus recirculation,[4] and drainage of mucoceles[5] are generally widely performed. In some clinics with appropriate tools and resources, limited primary sinus surgery and revision sinus surgeries are performed in the office setting.

Although the goals of treatment do not differ for patients undergoing in-office sinonasal procedures, patients undergoing office-based procedures must have realistic expectations and must accept that an office-based intervention may be more limited than a similar procedure undertaken in the operating room under general anesthesia. Patients must also be cautioned that additional procedures in the operating room may be required in the event of unexpected findings or in the situation where the procedure is unable to be completed in the awake patient.

MANAGEMENT OF ANXIETY AND PAIN

Patient comfort is critical not only to enhance the patient's experience but also to minimize anxiety. Pharmacologically, benzodiazepines, such as lorazepam at 1 to 2 mg given 1 hour before the procedure, are potent short-acting medications that can manage anxiety. However, there are several nonpharmacologic options. One such commercially available device, Nucalm (Solace Lifesciences, Inc, Wilmington, DE) is a clinical system that has four components to maximize relaxation and minimize anxiety: (1) a topical proprietary γ-aminobutyric acid cream to combat adrenaline, (2) cranial electrotherapy stimulation, (3) neuroacoustic soundtracks delivered via headphones, and (4) light-blocking eye masks designed to induce a state of deep relaxation. In a retrospective study, 25 patients undergoing sinus office procedures including total ethmoidectomy, inferior turbinate reductions, sphenoidotomy, and BCDs with the Nucalm system reported a reduction in anxiety post-procedure.[6]

Adequate anesthesia is critical to the success of the operation. A variety of local anesthetics is commercially available, and it is important to have a good understanding of each when considering their usage. Local anesthetics may be classified into esters and amides. Allergic reactions are uncommon but are slightly more likely to occur with the ester class of anesthetics. In general, local anesthetics act by blocking sodium channels, which prevents action potential propagation.

Rhinologic surgeons should be familiar with the toxicity profiles of local anesthetics. Burning or stinging may occur local to the administration site. If the local anesthetic is applied to the pharynx and/or oral cavity, suppression of the gag reflex is likely. Some patients also report difficulty swallowing or the sensation of throat blockage from numbing effect of the anesthetics on the pharynx. High plasma concentration initially produces central nervous system (CNS) stimulation (including seizures), followed by CNS depression (including respiratory arrest). The CNS stimulatory effect may be absent in some patients, particularly when amides are administered. Solutions that contain epinephrine may add to the CNS stimulatory effect. In addition, high plasma levels typically depress the heart and may result in bradycardia, arrhythmias, hypotension, cardiovascular collapse, and cardiac arrest. Local anesthetics that contain epinephrine may cause hypertension, tachycardia, and angina.

When selecting local anesthetics, it is important to consider their pharmacologic properties. Rate of onset, maximum dosage, and duration of effect are a few specific measures that can affect anesthetic choice. Lidocaine (amide) and tetracaine (ester) are two of the more common local anesthetics used in practice, and they have different pharmacologic properties. Lidocaine has a rapid rate of onset but has a short duration of action, whereas tetracaine has a slower rate of onset but provides a longer duration of action (**Table 1**). Most importantly, surgeons should be aware that a significantly smaller amount of tetracaine could lead to toxicity as compared with lidocaine.

A stepwise process helps to ensure that optimal anesthetic conditions are attained before the initiation of the procedure itself. Premedication with a short-acting benzodiazepine 1 hour before the procedure is considered on a case-by-case basis. Aerosolized oxymetazoline and 4% lidocaine are used for preliminary decongestion and anesthesia, respectively. Cottonoids soaked with 2% to 7% tetracaine or 4% lidocaine mixed with oxymetazoline are then placed within the middle meatus and in the nasal cavity under endoscopic visualization to ensure anesthetizing structures that may come in to contact with instruments during the procedure along with the treatment site. The cottonoids remain in place for approximately 15 to 20 minutes. Following this period, injection of 1% lidocaine with epinephrine (1:100,000) at involved sites is considered based on the procedure planned. Other techniques for local anesthesia have been described.[7]

One of the main benefits of office-based surgery is a reduction in recovery time because of the avoidance of general anesthesia. Recovery time is minimal for those undergoing office-based rhinology procedures. However, the lack of general anesthesia makes it even more critical that sufficient local anesthesia is provided to avoid significant levels of postoperatively pain. With proper topical and local anesthesia, most patients do not experience significant levels of pain and are managed with over-the-counter analgesics.

Table 1							
Pharmacology of lidocaine and tetracaine							
Drug	Onset	Max Dose, mg/kg		Max Dose, mg (70 kg)		Duration	
			With epi		With epi		With epi
Lidocaine	Rapid	4.5	7	315	490	120 min	240 min
Tetracaine	Slow	1.5	2.5	105	175	3 h	10 h

COMMON SINUS PROCEDURES
Balloon Catheter Dilation

The advent of BCD for the paranasal sinuses in the 2000s led to an explosion in office-based rhinologic surgery. Current patterns of use have suggested that the technology may be overused.[8–11] In response to the increased use of BCD, the American Academy of Otolaryngology–Head and Neck Surgery convened a working group to put forth a clinical consensus statement regarding balloon dilation of the sinuses.[12] The consensus statement was unable to delineate firm criteria for the use of BCD, but it did provide some general guidance on the appropriate and inappropriate uses of BCD (**Box 1**). The presence of polyps, a fungal ball, osteoneogenesis, or any suspicion of tumor are generally considered to be exclusions.

The basic technique of BCD involves a guide catheter, a guide wire, a BCD, and a manual pump mechanism to inflate and deflate the balloon. The process is based on Seldinger technique, where the guidewire is placed into the appropriate sinus, accurate placement is confirmed via illumination or navigation, and the balloon dilation catheter is advanced over the guidewire into the targeted ostium and expanded to 8 to 12 atm of pressure before being deflated and withdrawn. Only the transitional spaces of the maxillary ostium, sphenoid ostium, and frontal sinus outflow tract are targeted with BCD.

In-office BCD has been met with criticism associated with overuse; however, many studies, mainly industry sponsored, suggest high technical success rates, low complication rates, improvement in quality-of-life scores,[13–19] and even reductions in health

---

Box 1
Summary of clinical consensus statement: balloon dilation of the sinuses

BCD is not appropriate for patients without both sinonasal symptoms and positive findings on CT.

BCD is not appropriate for the management of headache in the absence of RARS or CRS.

BCD is not appropriate for the management of sleep apnea in the absence of RARS or CRS.

A preoperative CT scan is required before BCD is performed.

BCD is not appropriate for patients with sinonasal symptoms who do not demonstrate evidence of sinonasal disease on CT.

BCD is an adjunct to FESS in patients with CRSsNP.

There is a role for BCD in patients with persistent sinus disease who have had previous sinus surgery.

There is a role for BCD in managing patients with RARS as defined by the AAO-HNSF guideline based on symptoms and CT evidence of ostial occlusion and mucosal thickening.

FDA regulations regarding reuse of BCD devices should be followed.

BCD is performed in any setting as long as proper precautions and appropriate monitoring is performed.

BCD is performed under local anesthesia with or without sedation.

BCD improves short-term quality-of-life outcomes in patients with limited CRSsNP.

BCD is effective in frontal sinusitis.

Abbreviations: AAO-HNSF, American Academy of Otolaryngology–head and neck surgery foundation; CT, computed tomography; FDA, food and drug administration.

Adapted from Piccirillo J, Payne S, Rosenfeld R, et al. Clinical consensus statement: balloon dilation of the sinuses. Otolaryngol Head Neck Surg 2018;158(2):203–14; with permission.

care use[20] postoperatively. In cases of minimal CRS, traditional ESS and balloon may be options depending on the comfort of the operating surgeon.

Traditional Sinus Surgery Including Polypectomies

Led by BCD, the increase in office procedures also extends to include traditional ESS. As navigation systems with smaller footprints have found their way into the clinic setting, the range of sinuses and degree of polypectomy safely addressed in the office has expanded. Intervention with nonballoon instrumentation in cases of RARS, minimal CRSsNP, postoperative stenosis or synechiae, isolated fungal balls, and certain mucoceles are commonly accepted cases for the office setting. Additionally, the recurrence of polyps in CRS with polyposis is common and as such a means of addressing recurrent polyposis in the office setting is necessary. Polypectomies in this situation may be a method of reducing patient symptoms, improving topical medication delivery, and delaying or preventing the need for a formal revision surgery. The basic techniques of ESS and polypectomy are well known to practicing otolaryngologists and the nuances of such procedures are beyond the scope of this article.

Robust outcome data for in-office surgery are lacking. Scott and colleagues[21] reported on 315 patients undergoing traditional ESS under local anesthetic, which represents the largest series of patients undergoing traditional ESS in the office setting under local anesthetic that has been examined. They report a low complication rate and low revision rate.

Endoscopic Placement of Drug Delivery Implants

Sinuva (Intersect ENT, Menlo Park, CA) is a novel, high-dose, steroid-eluting implant now available for office placement in patients with recurrent polyposis who have previously undergone an ethmoidectomy. Using the delivery device provided with the implant, the surgeon places the implant into the ethmoid cavity, and the implant releases 1350 µg of mometasone furoate directly to the sinonasal mucosa over the span of 90 days. The procedure is straightforward. After an adequate delivery of local anesthesia and appropriate positioning of the patient, the insertion device is advanced as far into the ethmoid cavity as possible, and the implant is deployed. It expands on delivery, physically compressing the polyps and embedding itself in the ethmoid cavity (Video 1). Given that the device is roughly 7.5 mm in diameter, implantation may be challenging in patients with a narrow nasal or ethmoid cavity.

The outcome data are promising with results demonstrating improvement in nasal obstruction and smell at 30 days postimplantation and a reduction in polyp burden at 90 days postimplantation. Importantly, just over 60% of patients were no longer considered candidates for revision sinus surgery 90 days after undergoing implantation.[2] Longer-term results remain to be seen, and it is unclear if patients will need frequent implantation to maintain improvements. Additionally, health care cost analyses are needed to compare various treatment options for recurrent nasal polyps. Nonetheless, steroid-eluting implants with or without in-office polypectomies may allow the avoidance or at least delay in revision surgery in many patients.

Cryotherapy of Nasal Tissue

First described in 1970, cryotherapy to the sphenopalatine region within the nasal cavity resulted in significant improvements in nasal obstruction and reduction in nasal secretions. It was postulated that cryotherapy resulted in controlled necrosis with less collateral damage than other techniques, such as coagulation. Another advantage over competitive techniques, cryotherapy also targeted nerve endings rapidly providing concurrent pain control.[22,23]

Clarifix (Arrinex, Inc, Redwood City, CA), a Food and Drug Administration–approved device based on these initial experiences, provides delivery of cryotherapy to posterior nasal nerves within the posterior middle meatus. The procedure is simple to perform and well tolerated. After adequate delivery of local anesthesia and appropriate positioning of the patient, the balloon tip is placed into the posterior middle meatus under endoscopic visualization. The surgeon then manages a control dial that delivers nitrous oxide cryogen to the balloon tip for 30 seconds (Video 2).[3]

Cryosurgery of the posterior nasal tissue has been shown to be technically successful with a low complication rate. Additionally, total nasal symptom scores and rhinorrhea and nasal congestion scores were significantly reduced at all time points measured out to 1 year.[3] Limited data are available regarding the technology, but preliminary data are promising.

COMPLICATIONS

For any office-based sinonasal procedure, possible complications are similar to like procedures performed in the operating room. Given that patients are awake, additional complications of pain and anxiety may be experienced while undergoing the procedure. Additionally, there are the added risks of toxicity from topical anesthetics and of vasovagal syncope. Other possible complications include epistaxis, postoperative pain, scar, orbital and intracranial complications, or lack of significant improvement in symptoms.

The most common complication encountered by all these procedures is epistaxis. One must be fully prepared to manage epistaxis. Oxymetazoline- or epinephrine-soaked cottonoids should be on hand for all procedures. It would be wise to have monopolar or bipolar cautery devices available. Should severe epistaxis occur, the nose should be packed with cottonoids soaked with vasoconstrictors. This temporarily controls most bleeding aside from that occurring from large vessels. Suction cautery can then be used to coagulate any particular bleeding vessels encountered. Afterward, any number of topical procoagulants can be placed either directly over the area of concern or throughout the sinonasal cavity to prevent epistaxis recurrence postoperatively.

CODING, BILLING, AND REIMBURSEMENT

A complete review of rhinologic coding is beyond the scope of this article. However, in 2018, several changes were made to the sinonasal CPT codes. Because of the high frequency with which certain procedures were performed together, bundled codes were introduced for traditional ESS (31253, 31257, 31259) and for balloon procedures (31298). The valuations for the previous traditional ESS codes (31254-6, 31256, 31267, 31276, 31287-8) and balloon codes (31295-7) have also been adjusted.

Because of the high dose of steroids released from the steroid-eluting implants, these implants and future drug delivery devices are and may be treated as drugs rather than devices for billing purposes. There are two main strategies for billing: "buy and bill" directly, or purchasing the implant through a specialty pharmacy. If "buy and bill" is selected, the product is purchased by the physician directly, and the physician is responsible for obtaining authorization and submitting claims to insurance companies to be reimbursed. If one uses a specialty pharmacy, the pharmacy is responsible for obtaining authorization and billing for the drug delivery device. In this case, the physician only charges for services related to insertion.

Because cryotherapy of the posterior nasal nerve is a new technology, no specific CPT code is available for use. Some otolaryngologists are using CPT codes for similar procedures, whereas others are adopting a cash pay model.

SUMMARY

The ability to perform office-based rhinologic surgery is expanding at a rapid rate. The development of novel technologies is expanding the capabilities in this domain. Being able to target patients and pathologies that can be addressed in the office is critical to the successful implementation of in-office sinonasal surgery. These in-office procedures may reduce the burden of health care delivery by reducing recovery time and costs of procedures.

From a technical standpoint, the application of local anesthetic delivery is a crucial aspect of the procedure. With basic surgical skills, it is possible to use some of the newer technologies that are available in the office realm. However, to maximize the patient's ability to tolerate awake procedures, the practicing otolaryngologist must have sufficient surgical skill to perform procedures with little extraneous trauma.

Although the selection of patients and technical skills are essential to performing in-office rhinologic surgery, the otolaryngologist must always prioritize the needs of the patient. Office-based procedures can reduce the burden of health care delivery, but otolaryngologists must maintain the highest levels of integrity in situations that are often complicated by reimbursement incentives. When used responsibly, office-based sinonasal surgery is an effective method of treatment that may preclude the need for a formal operation in many patients and can play a significant role in reducing health care costs.

SUPPLEMENTARY DATA

Supplementary data to this article can be found online at https://doi.org/10.1016/j.otc. 2019.02.003.

REFERENCES

1. Gan EC, Habib AR, Hathorn I, et al. The efficacy and safety of an office-based polypectomy with a vacuum-powered microdebrider. Int Forum Allergy Rhinol 2013;3(11):890–5.
2. Kern RC, Stolovitzky J, Silvers S, et al. A phase 3 trial of mometasone furoate sinus implants for chronic sinusitis with recurrent nasal polyps. Int Forum Allergy Rhinol 2018;8(4):471–81.
3. Hwang PH, Lin B, Weiss R, et al. Cryosurgical posterior nasal tissue ablation for the treatment of rhinitis. Int Forum Allergy Rhinol 2017;7(10):952–6.
4. DelGaudio JM, Ochsner MC. Office surgery for paranasal sinus recirculation. Int Forum Allergy Rhinol 2015;5(4):326–8.
5. Barrow EM, DelGaudio JM. In-office drainage of sinus mucoceles: an alternative to operating-room drainage. Laryngoscope 2015;125(5):1043–7.
6. Marino M, Luong A, Yao W, et al. Nonpharmacologic relaxation technology for office-based rhinologic procedures. ORL J Otorhinolaryngol Relat Spec, in press.
7. Scott GM, Diamond C, Micomonaco DC. Assessment of a lateral nasal wall block technique for endoscopic sinus surgery under local anesthesia. Am J Rhinol Allergy 2018;32(4):318–22.
8. Svider P, Darlin S, Bobian M, et al. Evolving trends in sinus surgery: what is the impact of balloon sinus dilation? Laryngoscope 2018;128(6):1299–303.

9. Eloy JA, Svider PF, Bobian M, et al. Industry relationships are associated with performing a greater number of sinus balloon dilation procedures. Int Forum Allergy Rhinol 2017;7(9):878–83.

10. Calixto N, Gregg-Jaymes T, Liang J, et al. Sinus procedures in the Medicare population from 2000 to 2014: a recent balloon sinuplasty explosion. Laryngoscope 2017;127(9):1976–82.

11. Chaaban M, Baillargeon J, Baillargeon G, et al. Use of balloon sinuplasty in patients with chronic rhinosinusitis in the United States. Int Forum Allergy Rhinol 2017;7(6):600–8.

12. Piccirillo J, Payne S, Rosenfeld R, et al. Clinical consensus statement: balloon dilation of the sinuses. Otolaryngol Head Neck Surg 2018;158(2):203–14.

13. Cutler J, Truitt T, Atkins J, et al. First clinic experience: patient selection and outcomes for ostial dilation for chronic rhinosinusitis†. Int Forum Allergy Rhinol 2011; 1(6):460–5.

14. Stankiewicz JA, Truitt T, Atkins J, et al. Two-year results: transantral balloon dilation of the ethmoid infundibulum. Int Forum Allergy Rhinol 2012;2(3):199–206.

15. Sikand A, Silvers SL, Pasha R, et al. Office-based balloon sinus dilation: 1-year follow-up of a prospective, multicenter study. Ann Otol Rhinol Laryngol 2015; 124(8):630–7.

16. Karanfilov B, Silvers SL, Pasha R, et al. Office-based balloon sinus dilation: a prospective, multicenter study of 203 patients. Int Forum Allergy Rhinol 2013;3(5): 404–11.

17. Cutler J, Bikhazi N, Light J, et al. Standalone balloon dilation versus sinus surgery for chronic rhinosinusitis: a prospective, multicenter, randomized, controlled trial. Am J Rhinol Allergy 2013;27(5):416–22.

18. Bikhazi N, Light J, Schwartz M, et al. Standalone balloon dilation versus sinus surgery for chronic rhinosinusitis: a prospective, multicenter, randomized, controlled trial with 1-year follow up. Am J Rhinol Allergy 2014;28(4):323–9.

19. Chandra R, Kern R, Cutler J, et al. REMODEL larger cohort with long-term outcomes and meta-analysis of standalone balloon dilation studies. Laryngoscope 2016;126(1):44–50.

20. Levine S, Truitt T, Schwartz M, et al. In-office stand-alone balloon dilation of maxillary sinus ostia and ethmoid infundibula in adults with chronic or recurrent acute rhinosinusitis: a prospective, multi-institutional study with 1-year follow-up. Ann Otol Rhinol Laryngol 2013;122(11):665–71.

21. Scott J, Sowerby L, Rotenberg B. Office-based rhinologic surgery: a modern experience with operative techniques under local anesthetic. Am J Rhinol Allergy 2017;31(2):135–8.

22. Ozenberger JM. Cryosurgery in chronic rhinitis. Laryngoscope 1970;80(5): 723–34.

23. Ozenberger JM. Cryosurgery for the treatment of chronic rhinitis. Laryngoscope 1973;83(4):508–16.

In-office Functional Nasal Surgery

Richard Kao, MD[a], Cyrus C. Rabbani, MD[a], Jonathan Y. Ting, MD[b],
Taha Z. Shipchandler, MD[c],*

KEYWORDS

- Nasal surgery • Functional rhinoplasty • Nasal valve • In-office • Local anesthesia

KEY POINTS

- In-office nasal surgery should be considered for patients desiring immediate treatment without the adverse effects of general anesthesia, operating room costs, or scheduling delays.
- In-office nasal valve procedures are becoming more popular with more recent options available.
- Patient selection, preprocedure counseling, and effective local anesthesia are critical to ensuring patient satisfaction and outcomes.
- In-office inferior turbinoplasty using microdébrider, radiofrequency, ionized field ablation, and laser all have demonstrated effectiveness in the treatment of turbinate hypertrophy.
- In-office septoplasty may be considered in those with limited septal deflection or with bony or cartilaginous spur.

INTRODUCTION

Nasal airway obstruction is a common symptom encountered by the otolaryngologist. The investigation, diagnosis, and treatment of nasal airflow obstruction take time and patience. Numerous structural, immunologic, and disease processes have been associated with these symptoms. Septal deformity, nasal valve collapse/stenosis, and inferior turbinate hypertrophy top the list among anatomic and structural causes of nasal obstruction. Inevitably, the evaluation requires both thorough patient history and objective examination by a clinician.

Disclosures: Dr T.Z. Shipchandler is a member of the Speaker's Bureau for the Spirox Latera lateral nasal implant. Drs R. Kao, C.C. Rabbani, and J.Y. Ting have nothing to disclose.
[a] Department of Otolaryngology–Head and Neck Surgery, Indiana University School of Medicine, Indianapolis, IN, USA; [b] Division of Rhinology, Department of Otolaryngology–Head and Neck Surgery, Indiana University School of Medicine, Indianapolis, IN, USA; [c] Division of Facial Plastic, Aesthetic and Reconstructive Surgery, Department of Otolaryngology–Head and Neck Surgery, Indiana University School of Medicine, 1130 W. Michigan Street, Suite 400, Indianapolis, IN 46202, USA
* Corresponding author.
E-mail address: tshipcha@iupui.edu

Otolaryngol Clin N Am 52 (2019) 485–495
https://doi.org/10.1016/j.otc.2019.02.010
0030-6665/19/© 2019 Elsevier Inc. All rights reserved.

oto.theclinics.com

Static and dynamic structural weaknesses contribute to obstruction of the nasal airway. External nasal valve collapse takes place at the nasal ala and nostril, usually precipitated by deep inhalation. The internal nasal valve is described as the narrowest segment of the nasal airway with the highest contribution to overall nasal airway resistance. The valve boundaries are the anterior head of the inferior turbinate, septum, and caudal edge of the upper lateral cartilages. This narrow passage makes the internal valve vulnerable to multiple factors that may contribute to airway resistance and obstruction (eg, allergic rhinitis, septal deviation, and valve collapse).[1]

Ultimately, persistent nasal airway obstruction, despite medical and conservative therapy, generally prompts a discussion about surgical intervention. Effective surgical management is guided by patient symptoms, physical examination findings, and patient selection.

DIAGNOSIS

The introduction and improvements in nasal endoscopy have allowed thorough in-office evaluation. An evaluation of the nasal airway by endoscopy includes decongestion followed by investigation for valve narrowing, septal deviations, polyps, synechiae, tumors, and foreign bodies.

Although patients may find many ways to describe a symptom, one of the more common terms to relay nasal obstruction is nasal congestion. Medical treatment is the primary route of care for these patients, although, when ineffective, surgical options exist, including in-office procedures.

Septal deviations generally contribute to nasal obstruction, but they may not always be a major factor. Constantian and Clardy[2] revealed 54% of patients with subjectively obstructed nasal airway have a septum deviated to the side opposite the perceived obstruction. In these cases, the nasal valve may be the major contributor to obstruction. The nasal valve must be examined by both observed and forced breathing. External nasal valve collapse can be diagnosed by observing the nostril margin via basal view to determine the degree of alar collapse on moderate to deep inspiration through the nose. The Cottle and modified Cottle maneuver are well-described techniques for evaluating specific locations of valve collapse amenable to surgical therapy (**Fig. 1**). Other methods of objective assessment may include peak nasal inspiratory flow, acoustic rhinometry, and rhinometry. The utilization of these tests in the clinical setting is somewhat lacking given the time required. Surveys for symptoms are commonly used for assessment of nasal obstruction. The Nasal Obstruction Symptom Evaluation (NOSE) is a quality-of-life survey supported by an American Academy of Otolaryngology – Head and Neck Surgery consensus statement.[3] The visual analog scale also may be used as a surrogate for rhinomanometry, with adequate reliability.[4]

CONSIDERATIONS

Nasal obstruction can take a heavy toll on a patient's overall quality of life and daily productivity. In-office surgical procedures to address nasal airway obstruction generally avoid delays and recovery time by using minimally invasive techniques to achieve the goal of improved nasal airflow. Typically, patients drive themselves home or to work after such a procedure without any decrease in productivity.

Scott and colleagues[5] described a series of 315 in-office rhinologic procedures with an overall complication rate of 2.5%. These complications included pain, vasovagal episodes, bleeding, infection, and a swallowed pledget. An overall revision surgery

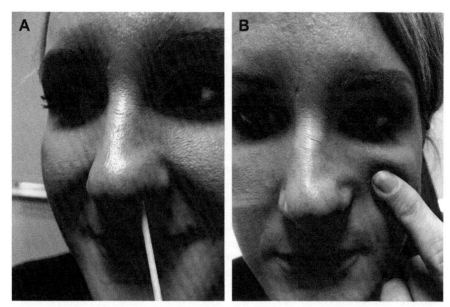

Fig. 1. (*A*) Cottle maneuver using cotton-tipped applicator to lateralize the lateral aspect of the nasal valve. (*B*) Modified Cottle maneuver to produce a similar effect to the Cottle maneuver.

rate of 11.7% was found for procedures, including turbinoplasty, endoscopic sinus surgery, septoplasty, rhinoplasty, and septorhinoplasty. Vasovagal responses to in-office procedures ranged from 0.16% to 0.6%. Many of these patients completed their procedure after a short recovery period.[5,6]

PATIENT SELECTION

In-office surgical procedures are not well suited for every patient; thus, determining who is a good candidate is critical. The nature and extent of the obstruction must be addressed. It is important that a patient's understanding and desires from intervention are well understood. There are patients who may elect a limited in-office procedure over a more extensive surgery in an operating room with general anesthesia despite a limited outcome.

Specifically, for in-office turbinate, nasal valve, and septum procedures, those patients who are medically unfit to undergo elective procedures due to the risks of general anesthesia should be considered. Coagulopathies and local anesthetic allergies should be known prior to initiating any office procedure. Patients on antiplatelet therapy may need to hold these medications if allowed by their cardiologist or other medical practitioners. The cardiovascular risks associated with holding antiplatelet or anticoagulant medications should be discussed both thoroughly with the surgeon and the cardiologist. Generally, aspirin is acceptable to continue whereas clopidogrel or ticagrelor should be held at least 5 days prior.

Patients must be aware of the cost of the procedure. There are large variations in insurance coverage when it comes to elective functional office nasal surgery. In-office nasal procedures may be denied, in which case the patient is expected to cover the procedural cost upfront. These charges should be honestly and openly discussed prior to any intervention.

ROOM SETUP AND PATIENT PREPARATION

The room in which these procedures are performed should be equipped with appropriate surgical equipment and lighting. Specifically, a headlight often is helpful for in-office nasal valve repair. Instruments should be laid accessible to both the assistant and surgeon along with supplementary anesthetic and topical vasoconstrictors. An electrocautery machine with appropriate tips may be stored within the office if necessary.

To improve patient comfort, the senior author (TZS) has speakers set up to play calming music at the patient's discretion. A low-dose anxiolytic, such as diazepam, alprazolam, or lorazepam, may be provided for mild sedation depending on the patient. It should be confirmed with patients that the position they remain in throughout the procedure not only is tolerable but comfortable. Patients typically are reclined to 45° for these procedures with a pillow under their knees and behind their head in the standard otolaryngology office examination chair. Local anesthetic of the nasal cavity requires a combination of topical and local injections. Topical agents generally contain an anesthetic and vasoconstriction component to achieve improved visualization and operative space. Topical spray with 1% phenylephrine and 4% lidocaine may be applied to start. Nasal pledgets then may be placed and soaked with 1 or more of the following: lidocaine, epinephrine, and tetracaine. Planned sites of incision and dissection are subsequently injected with lidocaine and diluted epinephrine with a 25-gauge needle (**Fig. 2**A). The patient generally may be observed for 30 minutes after the procedure to ensure recovery and hemostasis.

RHINOPLASTY AND NASAL VALVE REPAIR

Evaluation of the nasal valve comes down to distinguishing static and dynamic obstruction from either the upper or lower lateral cartilages. The Bernoulli principle states that as air velocity increases, the outward pressure decreases, leading to collapse from the sides of the nose. Weak lateral cartilage of the nose makes this collapse even more evident. The internal nasal valve accounts for approximately two-thirds of the total nasal airway resistance, and, with even a slight decrease in the cross-sectional area, symptomatic obstruction may arise.[7] On the other hand, static obstruction from nasal valve stenosis tends to remain at baseline regardless of the passage of air.

Worth noting are nonsurgical options for treatment of valve obstruction. Common commercial devices for nasal dilation include external nasal dilator strips, nasal stents,

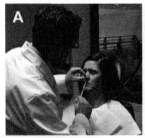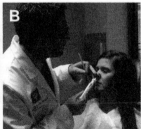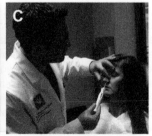

Fig. 2. (A) Patient receiving local anesthetic injection into left nasal sidewall in preparation for Latera implant. All images obtained for use with patient consent. (B) Insertion of the Latera implant using the delivery device. (C) After successful insertion of the implant, gentle pressure on the nasal bone is applied with a finger while pulling out the delivery device.

nasal clips, and septal stimulators. Limited data are available to support their use. A systematic review by Kiyohara and colleagues[8] found that external nasal dilators and nasal clips are the best studied and seem potential alternatives to surgical intervention. A reduction in nasal airway resistance was found with external nasal dilators (Breathe Right device, GlaxoSmithKline, Moon Township, PA, USA), and nose cones (Max-Air, Sanostec, Beverly Farms, MA, USA) were found to increase nasal airflow.[1,9]

Bioabsorbable Implant

As far as in-office treatment of nasal valve stenosis, few options exist that have gained significant popularity with more widespread use. One such implant is the Latera Bioabsorbable implant (Stryker, Kalamazoo, Michigan; **Fig. 3**). Latera has been available for more than 3 years, with data showing effectiveness 24 months from the procedure date, with improved NOSE scores absent adverse cosmetic changes. Latera can be placed either in the office using local anesthetic or in the operating room. The implant is bioabsorbable (poly-L-lactide and poly-D-lactide), thus resorbing on average 18 months after placement. The process the body undergoes to break down the implant leads to intrinsic stiffening of the nasal sidewall, thus giving a longlasting positive effect for the valve collapse even when the implant is no longer present. Latera is designed to serve as a sidewall and internal nasal valve support strut anchored caudally by the lateral crura of the lower lateral cartilage and cephalically by the sidewalls of the nasal bones. The implant is designed to rest in a plane just superficial to these structures in the sub-superficial musculoaponeurotic system (sub-SMAS) plane in the lateral sidewall, and also subperiosteally or just supraperiosteally on the nasal bones. This strut then supports and may even lateralize the sidewall of the nose, resulting in improved nasal breathing via decreased internal nasal valve collapse.

Latera comes prepackaged with 2 implants, a placement guide and a delivery device (see **Fig. 3**A). The placement guide is used to mark an area on the side of the nose where the perceived collapse is occurring (**Fig. 4**A, B). Great care must be taken to have the inferior edge of the implant cephalic to the alar-sidewall groove of the nose; otherwise, the impression of the implant may be visible and too close to the overlying dermis, causing potential inflammation or irritation. The implant is placed with relative ease under sterile conditions into the delivery device.

The senior author (TZS) has performed more than 170 Latera procedures with more than 30 in office under local anesthesia. They are well-tolerated procedures and

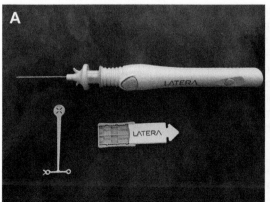
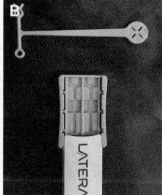

Fig. 3. (*A*) Latera implant device contents: 2 implants, placement guide, and delivery device. (*B*) Close-up photo of implants and placement guide.

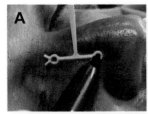
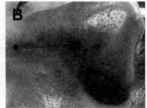
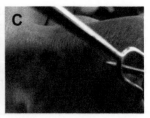

Fig. 4. (*A*) Use of the placement guide to mark the nasal side wall where perceived collapse is occurring. (*B*) Marks on the skin are used as guide for implant placement. (*C*) A double skin hook is used to apply downward traction, and the implant is placed between the 2 prongs of the skin hook using the marks as the intended implant position.

generally take 15 minutes to complete after a small room setup. Once the local anesthetic has been allowed to sit for 10 minutes, a double skin hook is used to apply traction downward on the nasal ala, with the 2 hooks placed in line on either side of where the intended implant will be placed (see **Fig. 4**C). Next, the implant is placed, taking great care to maintain the implant in the sub-SMAS plane stated previously (see **Fig. 2**B). Once the implant is in the nose, a finger is placed gently on the nasal bone while pulling out the delivery device (see **Fig. 2**C). This gentle finger pressure may aid in preventing the implant from coming back out with the delivery device.

The Latera device is among the earliest attempts to address the nasal valve while using a minimally invasive approach. It is recommended that a surgeon perform several procedures of this kind in the operating room before attempting this procedure in the office. In the authors' experience, thin-skinned individuals in the nasal bone region may show an impression of a visible implant, although this typically disappears within 4 weeks to 6 weeks. Extrusion of the implant through the skin is exceedingly rare and has not been experienced by the senior author (TZS), although it has been reported anecdotally generally due to superficial placement of the implant without persistent issues after removal. Other possible complications include no improvement from implant placement or retrieval of the implant from the nostril. Typically, a retrieval may occur early on when a surgeon is just gaining experience with the procedure.

The use of Latera is a suitable alternative for a patient who does not want the downtime of going to sleep for surgery or is medically unfit to receive a general anesthetic. If a patient has severe septal deviation and turbinate hypertrophy, Latera still may provide some improvement, but optimally the patient would be treated in the operating room with Latera and a concomitant septoplasty and/or turbinate reduction.

When evaluating a patient for Latera, it is important to note the skin thickness of the patient's nose in the nasal bone region. Otolaryngologists typically do not examine this area of skin. Very thin or crepe-like older skin in this area may show the impression of the implant, which may not be acceptable to a patient. In addition, if a patient wears glasses regularly, then the nose pieces of the glasses may rest on the superior edge of the Latera implant and cause some discomfort for the first several weeks after placement. It is important to discuss these issues with patient ahead of time.

Vestibular Skin Procedures

For the external nasal valve, a well-described rhinoplasty technique that may be suitable for an office setting is the lateral crural J-flap; this involves an incision over the lateral crus with excision of excess cartilage and vestibular skin.[5,10,11] An intranasal Z-plasty may be offered for internal/external nasal valve collapse; this is performed by removing portion of the vestibular skin with a skin Z-plasty performed at the site of valve collapse[12] (**Fig. 5**). In addition, Dolan and colleagues[13] describe a well-tolerated excision of 2 mm of mucosa, fibrous tissue, and caudal upper lateral cartilage with primary closure.

In an older patient with significant tip droop, weakened cartilages, and alar collapse, a rhinolift procedure may be considered. This procedure has been described as (1) an excision of redundant skin overlying the nasofrontal angle[14] and (2) a skin excision at the supratip crease with subsequent suspension of the lower lateral cartilages on the upper lateral cartilages.[15] Scott and colleagues[5] describe 4 septorhinoplasties performed with an external approach and septal cartilage grafting. Osteotomies have not been well described in the clinic setting, likely attributable to poor patient tolerance; however, closed nasal reduction after fracture may be suitable if addressed in a timely fashion.

Radiofrequency Remodeling

Recently, the Vivaer (Aerin Medical, Sunnyvale, California) was introduced as a low-frequency, nonablative, tissue remodeling device designed to address obstruction in the nasal valve region. The procedure is performed quickly in the office with injectable and/or topical anesthetic in the mucosal region of narrowing inside the nose. The device has shown promise to address an area not easily treated previously, specifically, the area just posterior to the nasal skin vestibule where the lateral wall is collapsing. Applying the tip of the device leads to remodeling and stiffening of the submucosal tissue and cartilage, thus opening the nasal airway.

INFERIOR TURBINATE HYPERTROPHY

The inferior turbinates play a key role in respiratory function and nasal physiology. Not only do they humidify, warm, and cleanse the air that is inspired through the nose, but also they contribute to inspiratory resistance, nasal defense system, and mucociliary transport.[16] Nasal obstruction often is caused by hypertrophic inferior turbinates, which may be caused by allergic or nonallergic rhinitis.[17] On examination, these patients most commonly present with pathologic mucosal inflammation.[18] Medical management is the first-line treatment, which includes the use of steroid sprays, antihistamines, decongestants, nasal saline sprays, and even immunotherapy in recalcitrant cases. In cases where medical management has failed, surgery may be indicated.

Surgical reduction of the inferior turbinates was introduced by Hartmann in the 1890s.[19] Total or partial turbinate resection was originally preferred, which had an increased risk of empty nose syndrome and atrophic rhinitis.[20] Submucous electrocautery was introduced for its quick and relatively bloodless method but produced

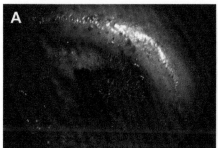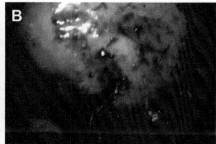

Fig. 5. (*A*) Z-plasty design within the left nasal vestibule via 0° endoscope. (*B*) Closer view of Z-plasty design via 0° endoscope.

temporary relief only, along with unwanted nasal dryness and edema. Similarly, cryotherapy offered a quick and bloodless option but caused diffuse mucosal injury due to the high surface area in contact with liquid nitrogen.

Over time, turbinoplasty as described by Mabry, has become a preferred surgical technique.[21] The goal of this surgery is to alleviate a patient's symptoms while preserving the mucosa and mucociliary function. As such, the turbinoplasty approach is characterized by raising a submucosal flap and resecting the hypertrophic submucosal tissues. The procedure is frequently supplemented with outward fracturing of the inferior turbinates, which is somewhat limited in the clinic setting due to comfort. Over time, multiple technologies have been introduced, each with its own strengths and weaknesses. Regardless of the method, multiple studies have demonstrated that the turbinoplasty approach provides the most lasting improvement in airway resistance.[22,23]

Radiofrequency-assisted Turbinoplasty

Radiofrequency (RF)-assisted turbinoplasty is a surgical procedure that uses RF heating to cause submucosal tissue destruction. RF has been used to reduce soft tissue volume in the soft palate and base of tongue in addition to the inferior turbinates. The device delivering this technology includes the Celon System (Olympus America, Melville, New York), which delivers 50 J to 70 J with a frequency of 470 Hz at a power setting of 15.[23] The Celon device has a bipolar probe needle measuring 1.3 mm in diameter with a protected tip, which aims to deliver the RF current to only its immediate vicinity. A previously described device in the literature of similar function is the Somnus (Somnus Medical, Sunnyvale, California).[22]

After application of topical anesthetic spray into the nasal cavity and local anesthetic injection into the turbinate, the tip is inserted into the head of the inferior turbinate under endoscopic visualization with a 0° endoscope. The tip is advanced posteriorly in the submucosal plane, parallel to turbinate's bony structure without exiting the turbinate. The instrument is then retracted anteriorly while using the coagulation setting so that a single continuous submucosal thermal lesion is created along the length of the inferior turbinate. The coagulation typically occurs over the span of 60 seconds to 90 seconds for each turbinate. Scar contraction occurs over the next 3 weeks, ultimately resulting in the decreased size of the inferior turbinates Celon System (Olympus America, Melville, New York).

This method of turbinate reduction offers a relatively easy setup and preparation. Patients typically are able to return to normal activity levels after the procedure and typically have high patient comfort and satisfaction.

Ionized Field Ablation-assisted Turbinoplasty

The concept of ionized field ablation centers on its use of a RF-activated plasma to resect tissue. Its electrodes are configured in a specific fashion to create a plasma field of ionized sodium molecules, which ablate tissues while dispersing minimal excess heat energy in that process. The most commonly used device delivering this technique is aptly named cold ablation (Smith & Nephew, Texas) after its so-called cold ablation. The thermal effect of the process is approximately 45°C to 85°C, significantly lower than traditional RF techniques. It has numerous applications in the head and neck, including ablation and resection of tissues in the oral cavity, oropharynx, and nasopharynx, airway, and paranasal sinuses.

The more recently developed Turbinator wand (Smith & Nephew) used with coblation technology incorporates suction into the handpiece, which provides a more visible removal of submucosal tissue intraoperatively. Although the wand is significantly larger at 2.9 mm in width, it removes tissue more aggressively and provides improved hemostasis than older coblation techniques. A preliminary study reveals good outcomes, not inferior to microdébrider-assisted methods.[24]

Microdébrider-assisted Turbinoplasty

Microdébrider-assisted turbinoplasty has emerged as a popular technique due to the familiarity with the technology, which is frequently used in endoscopic sinus surgery. The inferior turbinate blade uses an elevated, rotating, oscillating tip that removes obstructive tissue in a cold steel fashion. Saline irrigation and suction are incorporated into this device to clear the tip of debris and actively extract the tissue excised from the surgical site.

To provide access to the turbinate, a stab incision is often made at the head of the turbinate and a submucosal plane is developed. The turbinate blade can then be advanced through this plane with ease to begin resecting tissue. The blade may be rotated to address different areas of obstruction, while care is taken to not perforate through the posterior turbinate mucosa. A more invasive extension of this technique uses a submucosal resection of some portion of the turbinate bone in addition to its soft tissue.[20]

The use of microdébrider requires a comparably more involved setup, which includes saline irrigation and suction simultaneously. As a result, proper function relies on these constituents working correctly as well. Due to the cold blade resection, there is increased risk for postoperative bleeding than with thermoablative techniques.

A meta-analysis of 1523 cases from 26 studies comparing these methods showed that all the methods (RF and coblation grouped together vs microdébrider) produced significant symptomatic relief, with no significant difference in the visual analog scale or rhinomanometry postoperatively.[22] There were insufficient data to conclude whether concurrent out-fracturing provided any additional benefit. Two high-quality prospective and randomized studies included in this analysis revealed that microdébrider-assisted turbinoplasty was statistically favored in providing symptom relief[17] and providing longer-lasting effects over 6 months postoperatively.[25]

Senior Author's Choice for In-office Turbinate Reduction

The senior author's (TZS) prefers the coblation technique for in-office turbinate reduction mainly due to the ease of setup and patient tolerance. The risk of bleeding is very low compared with the cold techniques of submucosal resection, which may lead to patients experiencing anterior bleeding from their nose and down their throat during the procedure. Coblation is also an easy setup with minimal equipment necessary compared with formal submucosal resection with microdébrider. Lastly, coblation, due to its lower thermal heat level, causes less pain during and after the procedure compared with RF. Tolerance and ease of setup, therefore, are the driving forces for the author's choice of coblation for in-office turbinate reduction.

SEPTOPLASTY

In-office septoplasty can be performed under local anesthetic in a fashion similar to that in the operating room. The ideal patient for this procedure is one with limited cartilaginous deviation or an isolated spur, such that precise surgical resection can greatly improve a patient's symptoms.[26] In the instance of septal deviation, the procedure follows the standard operation performed in the operating room using open or endoscopic visualization. Special attention is given to properly anesthetize all the intended areas of resection along the septum as well as the hemitransfixion site.

Ensuring patient comfort during in-office septoplasty is of utmost consideration, especially because the comfortable patient is more likely to stay still during the procedure.

SUMMARY

Surgical procedures in the office require a prepared clinician and patient. There are a growing number of techniques to treat patients for nasal airway obstruction. Although not all patients are suited for an in-office functional nasal airway procedure, there are many potentially favorable candidates. Beyond the cost-saving benefits, consider performing in-office functional nasal surgery in patients with desire for limited surgical interventions or those who are medically unfit for general anesthesia should be considered.

REFERENCES

1. Portugal LG, Mehta RH, Smith BE, et al. Objective assessment of the breathe-right device during exercise in adult males. Am J Rhinol 1997;11:393–7.
2. Constantian MB, Clardy RB. The relative importance of septal and nasal valvular surgery in correcting airway obstruction in primary and secondary rhinoplasty. Plast Reconstr Surg 1996;98:38–54 [discussion: 55–8].
3. Stewart MG, Smith TL, Weaver EM, et al. Outcomes after nasal septoplasty: results from the Nasal Obstruction Septoplasty Effectiveness (NOSE) study. Otolaryngol Head Neck Surg 2004;130:283–90.
4. Ciprandi G, Mora F, Cassano M, et al. Visual analog scale (VAS) and nasal obstruction in persistent allergic rhinitis. Otolaryngol Head Neck Surg 2009; 141:527–9.
5. Scott JR, Sowerby LJ, Rotenberg BW. Office-based rhinologic surgery: a modern experience with operative techniques under local anesthetic. Am J Rhinol Allergy 2017;31:135–8.
6. Radvansky BM, Husain Q, Cherla DV, et al. In-office vasovagal response after rhinologic manipulation. Int Forum Allergy Rhinol 2013;3:510–4.
7. Haight JS, Cole P. The site and function of the nasal valve. Laryngoscope 1983; 93:49–55.
8. Kiyohara N, Badger C, Tjoa T, et al. A comparison of over-the-counter mechanical nasal dilators: a systematic review. JAMA Facial Plast Surg 2016;18:385–9.
9. Raudenbush B. Stenting the nasal airway for maximizing inspiratory airflow: internal Max-Air Nose Cones versus external Breathe Right strip. Am J Rhinol Allergy 2011;25:249–51.
10. O'Halloran LR. The lateral crural J-flap repair of nasal valve collapse. Otolaryngol Head Neck Surg 2003;128:640–9.
11. Tan S, Rotenberg B. Functional outcomes after lateral crural J-flap repair of external nasal valve collapse. Ann Otol Rhinol Laryngol 2012;121:16–20.
12. Dutton JM, Neidich MJ. Intranasal Z-plasty for internal nasal valve collapse. Arch Facial Plast Surg 2008;10:164–8.
13. Dolan RW, Catalano PJ, Innis W, et al. In-office surgical repair of nasal valve stenosis. Am J Rhinol Allergy 2009;23:111–4.
14. Kabaker SS. An adjunctive technique to rhinoplasty of the aging nose. Head Neck Surg 1980;2:276–81.
15. Hu M. External approach for the treatment of the aging nasal tip. Int J Head Neck Surg 2016;7:165–7.

16. Lee KC, Hwang PH, Kingdom TT. Surgical management of inferior turbinate hypertrophy in the office: three mucosal sparing techniques. Oper Tech Otolayngol Head Neck Surg 2001;12:107–11.

17. Liu CM, Tan CD, Lee FP, et al. Microdebrider-assisted versus radiofrequency-assisted inferior turbinoplasty. Laryngoscope 2009;119:414–8.

18. Siegel GJ, Seiberling KA, Haines KG, et al. Office CO2 laser turbinoplasty. Ear Nose Throat J 2008;87:386–90.

19. Maskell S, Eze N, Patel P, et al. Laser inferior turbinectomy under local anaesthetic: a well tolerated out-patient procedure. J Laryngol Otol 2007;121:957–61.

20. Janda P, Sroka R, Baumgartner R, et al. Laser treatment of hyperplastic inferior nasal turbinates: a review. Lasers Surg Med 2001;28:404–13.

21. Veit JA, Nordmann M, Dietz B, et al. Three different turbinoplasty techniques combined with septoplasty: prospective randomized trial. Laryngoscope 2017; 127:303–8.

22. Acevedo JL, Camacho M, Brietzke SE. Radiofrequency ablation turbinoplasty versus microdebrider-assisted turbinoplasty: a systematic review and meta-analysis. Otolaryngol Head Neck Surg 2015;153:951–6.

23. Gouveris H, Nousia C, Giatromanolaki A, et al. Inferior nasal turbinate wound healing after submucosal radiofrequency tissue ablation and monopolar electrocautery: histologic study in a sheep model. Laryngoscope 2010;120:1453–9.

24. Khong GC, Lazarova L, Bartolo A, et al. Introducing the new Coblation Turbinator turbinate reduction wand: our initial experience of twenty-two patients requiring surgery for nasal obstruction. Clin Otolaryngol 2018;43:382–5.

25. Lee JY, Lee JD. Comparative study on the long-term effectiveness between coblation- and microdebrider-assisted partial turbinoplasty. Laryngoscope 2006;116:729–34.

26. Thamboo A, Patel ZM. Office procedures in refractory chronic rhinosinusitis. Otolaryngol Clin North Am 2017;50:113–28.

Office-Based Otology Procedures

Manuela Fina, MD*, Douglas Chieffe, MD

KEYWORDS

- Office-based otology • Endoscopic ear surgery • Myringoplasty
- Intratympanic injection

KEY POINTS

- The scope of office-based otologic procedures has broadened with the incorporation of endoscopic techniques.
- Endoscopy is particularly useful to inspect anterior perforations, retraction pockets and ears with narrow or stenotic ear canals.
- Use of endoscopy allows inspection of deep retraction pockets whose depth cannot be fully visualized under microscopy, potentially modifying the criteria for surgical intervention.
- Repair of simple, uncomplicated tympanic perforations can be performed in-office using autologous or heterologous tissue-engineered grafts.
- Intratympanic injections are an effective, low-risk options for the treatment of sudden sensorineural hearing loss and intractable Meniere's Disease.

 Video content accompanies this article at http://www.oto.theclinics.com.

INTRODUCTION

Of the otolaryngology subspecialties, otology may appear as the field with the fewest innovations in the office-based setting. One may think that the otology practice remains centered on the microscopic ear examination, cerumen cleaning, mastoid debridement, myringotomy with tube placement, and fat graft myringoplasty. However, new optics, high-definition digital monitors, tissue-engineered grafts, and evidence-based protocols for transtympanic perfusions have entered the contemporary office practice of otology, not only changing the way we treat common otologic problems but also the way we select patients for surgical intervention.

Disclosure: Both authors have no conflicts of interest or financial ties to disclose.
Department of Otolaryngology, University of Minnesota, Minneapolis, MN, USA
* Corresponding author. Department of Otolaryngology, 420 Delaware Street Southeast, MMC 396, Minneapolis, MN 55455.
E-mail address: finax003@umn.edu

Otolaryngol Clin N Am 52 (2019) 497–507
https://doi.org/10.1016/j.otc.2019.02.004
0030-6665/19/© 2019 Elsevier Inc. All rights reserved.

The objective of this article is to describe the most recent innovations in office-based otologic procedures for the treatment of the most common otologic conditions.

IN-OFFICE OTOENDOSCOPY

Traditionally, the microscope is considered the tool of choice to examine the tympanic membrane. In the past decade, endoscopes have been incorporated by otologic surgeons as an important adjunct tool not only in the surgical setting but also in office practices.

The wider angle of view and high-quality image provided by otoendoscopy allows the visualization of certain pathologies, the examination of which is challenging under microscopy. Endoscopy increases the ability to inspect the depth of retraction pockets, potentially changing the indication for surgical intervention. Similarly, the ability to visualize a very anteriorly based tympanic perforation can change the criteria for in-office myringoplasty.

Choice of Endoscopes for the Office

The first endoscopes used specifically for otoscopy were short, rigid scopes 6 cm in length. These short endoscopes are useful for the inspection and photographic documentation of the tympanic membrane. However, their use in office-based otologic procedures is limited because the short shaft places the camera hand in the way of the instrument hand. Longer endoscopes allow the surgeon's hands to be staggered so that procedures can be performed without hand collision.

In our office, we prefer rigid sinus scopes (Karl Storz Endoscopy-America, El Segundo, CA) 16 cm in length and 4 mm in diameter to inspect the tympanic membrane as they are already common tools for sinus endoscopy. For most ear examinations, 0-degree endoscopes are used; 30-degree endoscopes are useful for visualization of retraction pockets and inspection of anterior tympanic membrane perforations obscured by a prominent anterior canal wall. Pediatric rigid sinus scopes 2.7 mm in diameter and 16 cm in length are used for narrow ear canals, exostosis, or pediatric ear examinations. In the author's experience, children as young as 3 years of age have been cooperative in allowing endoscopic ear examination by being allowed to watch the screen. The endoscope is connected through the light source to a camera and to a high-definition screen monitor.

Patient Positioning

The otoendoscopic examination is best performed with the patient slightly reclined in the examining chair and the surgeon in a sitting position. The screen monitor is positioned directly across from the surgeon and at a close distance to avoid strain from neck turning (**Fig. 1**).

Endoscopic Examination of Retraction Pockets

Traditionally, the distinction between retraction pocket and cholesteatoma has been based on microscopic examination. Retraction pockets can be classified from grade 0 through V for pars flaccida retraction and from grade I through IV for pars tensa retraction.[1,2]

Currently, the decision to recommend surgery is a clinical judgment based on the microscopic examination and radiologic findings. Retraction pockets whose debris cannot be fully cleaned and whose depth cannot be visualized fulfill the definition of cholesteatoma and should be surgically explored.[3]

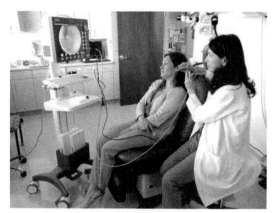

Fig. 1. In-office otoendoscopy setup with a Karl Storz Telepak unit. (*Courtesy of* Karl Storz Endoscopy-America, El Segundo, CA, ©2018; with permission.)

The progressive use of endoscopes in the otologic setting will eventually change our parameters to surgically intervene. The endoscopic inspection of retraction pockets provides an expanded view of the depth of the retraction beyond the scutum. Thus, deep retraction pockets can be fully monitored under endoscopy and may no longer fit the current criteria for surgical intervention.

A clean pars tensa retraction with development of myringo-stapediopexy with limited conductive hearing loss can be followed clinically (**Fig. 2**, Video 1). Similarly very extensive, grade V pars flaccida retraction with a wide orifice and exposure of the head and neck of the malleus and no evidence of keratin accumulation can also be observed clinically (**Fig. 3**).

As endoscopic proficiency is gained, it is possible not only to inspect but also to suction and clean debris within a retraction pocket not accessible with the microscope. This is particularly useful in the setting of an epitympanic retraction with a very narrow ear canal or a mesotympanic retraction with a prominent scutum.

Endoscopic Examination of Tympanic Perforations

Pre-operative endoscopy of tympanic perforations provides important information for surgical planning. Many perforations are small in size, but full visualization may not be

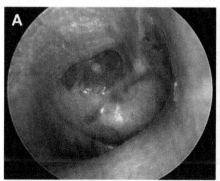
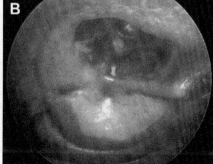

Fig. 2. Pars tensa retraction with incus erosion and myringo-stapediopexy examined with 0-degree (*A*) and 30-degree (*B*) scopes.

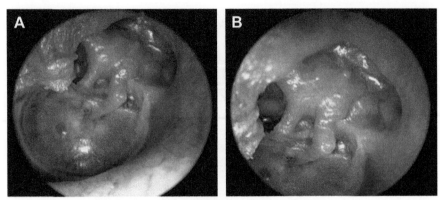

Fig. 3. Extensive grade V pars flaccida retraction of the right ear examined with 0-degree (*A*) and 30-degree (*B*) rigid scopes.

possible under microscopy because of an anterior canal bulge or a prominent tragus. Endoscopy offers the advantage of visualizing the anterior tympanic annulus and the entire margin of the perforation.

For posterior tympanic perforations, endoscopy can provide useful information on the status of the ossicular chain. A 30-degree endoscope angled in the posterior aspect of the perforation can reveal erosion or tapering of the long process of the incus or presence of epithelium adherent to the ossicles. Epithelial migration under the medial surface of the tympanic membrane may be overlooked under microscopic examination but may be detected by advancing the endoscope close to the perforation. The detection of such findings pre-operatively are extremely important when counseling the patient for surgery, as any otologic surgeon with experience knows how an apparently innocent looking tympanic perforation may reveal occult cholesteatoma or unexpected ossicular discontinuity.

In-Office Transtympanic Middle Ear Endoscopy

Transtympanic middle ear endoscopy requires much thinner endoscopes to be inserted in the middle ear cavity through a small myringotomy. Endoscopes 2 mm in diameter are used. This surgical technique has been described to inspect the middle ear space for ossicular chain pathology, presence of cholesteatoma in the middle ear cavity, and perilymphatic fistula.[4,5] The endoscopic detection and removal of obliterative fibrous tissue over the round window in patients refractory to transtympanic perfusion for Meniere's disease has been described as well.[6]

In-Office Endoscopic Examination of Post-surgical Results

Endoscopy is an excellent way to document and follow post-operative healing. Photography does not replace the need for a thorough and concise description of the physical examination in the patient record, but adding photographs to progress notes makes this nearly foolproof. This is especially useful in practices in which a patient may see multiple providers.

Another advantage of otoendoscopy is the wide-angled view of the external ear canal that is otherwise covered by the speculum under microscopy. Small post-operative inclusion pearls along the posterior ear canal can be missed under microscopic examination and, if not detected and enucleated, may progress to canal cholesteatoma. Another more unusual complication that can be obscured by the speculum is the development of a sinus tract between the site of the transcanal incision and the mastoidectomy cavity. These cases typically present with intermittent drainage and no obvious source seen on the tympanic membrane.

Endoscopic Inspection and Debridement of Mastoid Cavities

Every surgeon knows the challenges of debriding a mastoid cavity with a small, stenotic meatoplasty or a mastoid cavity with a high facial ridge and low tegmen. Endoscopic examination of challenging mastoid cavities may reveal areas of granulation tissue, mucositis, or recurrent cholesteatoma in previously hidden areas. With the endoscope in the non-dominant hand and an instrument in the dominant hand, the cavity can be inspected, debrided and suctioned, and granulation tissue cauterized.

High-Definition Digital Monitors, Data Management, and Digital Photodocumentation

When included in a patient's chart, serial photography taken during office visits can be useful to compare the size of perforations and retraction pockets over time. It is important to develop a consistent methodology when taking photographs of the ear, as the angle and lighting can make a difference in the assessment of size and depth of the pathologic ear findings. The size of the tympanic membrane perforation can be deceiving even under endoscopic examination. Because of the oblique position of the tympanic membrane in the ear canal, perforations are often viewed from an angle, making them seem smaller.

The ability to show patients their ear on a screen is an indispensable tool when counseling patients on the need for surgery. There is no better visual aid than a photograph of the patient's ear. Endoscopy can also present good teaching opportunities for students and residents, as anatomy and pathology can be easily pointed out on the screen.

The use of endoscopy in the clinic does not stop at examination and documentation; it can also be used as the primary tool to repair tympanic membrane perforations.

IN-OFFICE ENDOSCOPIC MYRINGOPLASTY
Indications and Patient Selection

We define office-based myringoplasty as the transcanal repair of tympanic membrane defects without the use of sedation or general anesthesia and without elevation of a tympanomeatal flap. Because of the delicate manipulation of the tympanic membrane, not all adult patients may be comfortable or cooperative enough to undergo repair under straight local anesthesia. For the same reason, general anesthesia is recommended for younger patients.

Traditionally, indications for in-office myringoplasty have been limited to small, dry perforations, the margins of which are fully visible under microscopic examination. The inability to visualize the anterior margin can preclude not just the in-office repair but even a transcanal microscopic approach under general anesthesia and may require a posterior auricular approach. Endoscopy improves visualization of the anterior rim of the tympanic membrane, thus expanding the indications for in-office myringoplasty for anterior perforations the margins of which are not fully visible under microscopic technique.

Marginal perforations, wet perforations, and suspected ossicular pathology are better suited for tympanoplasty under general anesthesia with elevation of a tympanomeatal flap and middle ear exploration.

A relative contraindication to in-office repair is the presence of extensive myringo-sclerosis. Thick plaques may be lined by thin atrophic epithelium and may require extensive excision that is more appropriately performed under general anesthesia.

In general, perforations less than 25% to 30% can be repaired in the office; however, some authors report success with larger perforations.[7] Larger perforations require not only a larger graft but also more complex underlay techniques to prevent graft displacement or graft failure. In addition, larger size perforation cannot be adequately repaired solely with a fat patch because of the tendency for fat to reabsorb or to possibly displace in the middle ear space.

There are few reports of long-term results after in-office myringoplasty; however, with appropriate patient selection, most closure results are reported around 80% to 90%, which is comparable with outcomes of tympanoplasty performed under general anesthesia and with elevation of a tympanomeatal flap.[8] In the senior author's practice, endoscopy has facilitated a shift toward repairing more perforations in the office.

Choice of Graft Materials

In addition to fat, cartilage, and fascia grafts, new tissue-engineered grafts such as porcine small intestinal submucosa (SIS) (Biodesign; Cook Biotech, West Lafeyette, IN) and hyaluronic acid discs (Epidisc Otologic Lamina; Medtronic, Jacksonville, FL) are available.

In the senior author's experience, the use of porcine SIS grafts has provided similar results to those of fat myringoplasty, with the advantage of avoiding an external incision and decreasing post-operative pain. In addition, this tissue-engineered material is embedded in fibroblast growth factor, which promotes graft revascularization. Furthermore, its acellular composition results in a transparent appearance of the healed graft (**Figs. 4** and **5**). We limit the use of SIS to perforations less than 30% in size. Early results of myringoplasty using porcine SIS have shown comparable results with autologous fascia grafts.[9,10] Hyaluronic acid discs placed as an overlay over fat myringoplasty have also shown good results.[8]

For patients with perforations greater than 30%, or in those with objections to porcine-based materials, we place a composite cartilage-perichondrium button graft (Video 2).

Methods and Surgical Technique

Written informed consent is obtained and the patient is positioned supine with the head slightly elevated. The outer ear canal is prepped with betadine and the ear is draped with surgical towels. Optimal hemostasis and the administration of local anesthesia is essential for the success of the procedure. The ear canal is injected with 2 mL

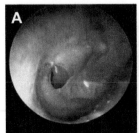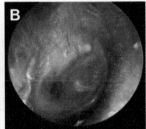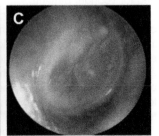

Fig. 4. Porcine small intestinal submucosa myringoplasty: pre-operative (*A*), 10-week post-operative (*B*), and 6 months post-operative(*C*).

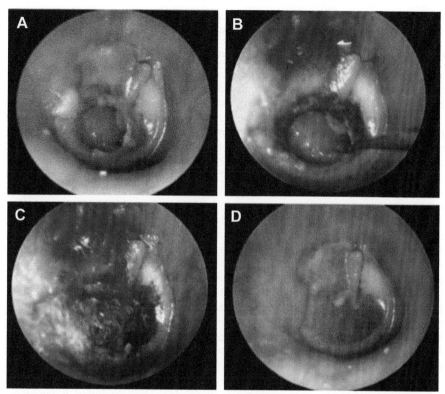

Fig. 5. Porcine small intestinal submucosa myringoplasty: pre-operative examination (*A*), rimming of perforation margins (*B*), inset as an inlay (*C*), and 3 months post-operative (*D*).

of 1% lidocaine with 1:100,000 epinephrine. Blanching of the tympanic membrane indicates adequate infiltration of the anesthetic. Extreme care is used to avoid leaking of anesthetic solution into the middle ear, as this can result in post-operative vertigo. It is advisable to wait 10 minutes before beginning to ensure that the anesthetic has appropriately infiltrated the tissue. The screen monitor is placed directly across from the surgeon so that the surgeon can easily see the screen without straining the neck. This also allows the patient to observe the procedure and reinforces the importance of not moving their head. For most cases, a 0-degree rigid endoscope of 4 mm diameter is sufficient for visualization of the perforation margins. Narrow ear canals may require a pediatric 4-mm rigid sinus scope, and very anterior perforations may require a 30-degree angled scope.

The perforation is then gently de-epithelialized circumferentially by teasing the margins with a Rosen needle and everting the margins outward, stripping less tissue than with a postage-stamping technique.

Fat grafts are positioned as a dumbbell across the perforation. Cartilage button grafts are harvested via a small incision in the tragus or the conchal bowl. A disposable skin punch (3, 4, or 5 mm) may be used to cut a disc-shaped graft 1 mm larger than the perforation. The graft is harvested along with perichondrium. A groove is cut in the edge of the cartilage and the graft is positioned with the perichondrium laterally and the tympanic membrane in the cut groove (see Video 2).

When utilizing porcine SIS, a small piece of Gelfoam is placed in the middle ear to support the graft. The porcine SIS graft is cut into 2 discs of slightly larger dimensions than the size of the perforation. One disc is placed medially to the perforation and the second disc is placed laterally. This sandwich-type scaffold favors epithelial regrowth.

Role of Nasal Endoscopy in the Contemporary Otology Practice

In today's office-based practice, the otologist has been trained to perform flexible naso-pharyngo-laryngoscopy in patients with ear pain and/or adult onset of otitis media with effusion to rule out upper airway malignancy or nasopharyngeal masses as a cause of referred otalgia or middle ear effusions. Traditionally, chronic pathologies of the ear such as chronic suppurative otitis media with perforation, cholesteatoma, or chronic otitis media with retraction are not considered routine indications for nasal endoscopy. However, new studies on the role of the eustachian tube (ET) in the pathogenesis of chronic ear disease and new ET dilation techniques are changing the way we approach and examine patients with chronic ear disease.[11] In patients with chronic ear conditions, nasopharyngoscopy has an important diagnostic role.

Adult onset of chronic mucoid otitis media is often related to chronic sinus pathologies affecting the respiratory epithelium of both middle ear and paranasal sinuses, and warrants nasal endoscopy to diagnose and treat possible concomitant sinus pathology.[12] Nasopharyngoscopy may also reveal a pathology localized to the ET orifice. Inspection of the ET orifices may reveal collapsed, narrow, edematous, or lymphoid hyperplastic appearance. Nasopharyngoscopy may reveal mulberry hypertrophy of the inferior turbinates directly obstructing the ET lumen, obstructive adenoid hypertrophy, or unexpected synechiae from previous adenoidectomy scars restricting opening of the ET orifice. Nasopharyngoscopy in the setting of atrophic pars tensa atelectasis may reveal patulous ET. In these patients habitual sniffing to alleviate ear symptoms resulted in chronic atelectasis and an ET dilation procedure would be contraindicated.

In sum, the role of nasopharyngoscopy for the otologist has expanded. A careful examination of the nasopharynx and ET orifice is an essential part of the complete otologic examination in patients with chronic ear pathologies.

TRANSTYMPANIC INNER EAR PERFUSION

Transtympanic perfusion permits drug delivery directly to the middle and inner ear structures. After instillation in the middle ear, drugs pass through the round window membrane and oval window annular ligament, and diffuse throughout the perilymph and endolymph.[13] This can achieve high concentrations of the drug within the cochlea and vestibular apparatus while avoiding systemic side effects. In-office intratympanic (IT) injections are used for the treatment of sudden sensorineural hearing loss and refractory Meniere's disease. Despite innumerable trials, there is no consensus on the optimal regimen for either disease.

INTRATYMPANIC STEROID INJECTIONS FOR TREATMENT OF SUDDEN SENSORINEURIAL HEARING LOSS
Indications and Patient Selection

For patients with confirmed sudden sensorineural hearing loss, initiation of either oral or IT steroids is recommended as a rescue therapy. IT steroids are indicated for those patients who cannot tolerate systemic steroids or for those patients who have not responded to oral steroids.[14] Recent studies have demonstrated non-inferiority in hearing recovery between oral and IT steroids.[15] Intratympanic steroids have more focal side effects—pain (27%), transient vertigo 27%, tympanic membrane perforations (3.9%), and otitis media (4.7%)—compared with oral steroids.

Sudden profound sensorineural hearing loss carries a poor prognosis for hearing recovery.[16] For these cases we recommend simultaneous oral and IT steroid injection to maximize all the possible chances for hearing recuperation.[17] Although many studies exclude patients with onset of symptoms greater than 2 weeks, we treat patients up to 4 weeks after symptom onset. If the patient has less than complete recovery with oral steroids, we then offer the IT steroid injections modality as a salvage.

Surgical Technique and Dosage

After obtaining informed consent, the patient is positioned supine with the head elevated 30° and the neck turned with the affected ear facing upward. Topical phenol 89% (Apdyne Phenol Applicator Kit; Apdyne Medical, Denver, CO) is used to provide anesthesia to the posterior inferior quadrant of the tympanic membrane. A pressure-release puncture hole is first made using a tuberculin syringe with a 1.5-inch-long 25-gauge needle. Using the same needle and syringe, 0.4 mL of 40 mg/mL methylprednisolone is injected just inferior to the release hole. Because of the small volume of the middle ear space and the patient tendency for swallowing, we inject 0.2 mL into the middle ear followed by an additional 0.2 mL 15 minutes later. The patient is instructed to remain in the same position for 30 minutes and to avoid frequent swallowing. The patient is assessed for vertigo before discharging home with follow-up arranged for the next 3 injections, performed twice weekly. An audiogram is obtained 1 week after the fourth and final injection to assess improvement and discuss further evaluation of their sudden SNHL if not already completed.

Choice of Steroid Solution (Methylprednisolone versus Dexamethasone)

Initially, methylprednisolone (MP) was preferred over dexamethasone (DX) after one animal pharmacokinetic study showed higher and more prolonged levels of MP in the endo- and perilymph.[18] However, subsequent studies have shown no difference in recovery rates between IT DX and IT MP when used for primary treatment.[19] Methylprednisolone has shown to cause more pain and burning than DX.[19] However, given the inconclusive evidence, the choice of steroid is physician dependent.

Intratympanic injections for treatment of Meniere's disease

For Meniere's disease refractory to diuretics and salt restriction, intra-tympanic steroid injections may be offered as a minimally invasive, vestibular-sparing treatment. The exact mechanism of action is unknown, and, because there are few high-quality studies, the benefit is similarly unknown.[20] However, given the low side-effect profile and potential for benefit, IT steroids have been used in the treatment of Meniere's disease refractory to medical treatment.[21] If IT steroid injections fail, vestibular-sparing surgery (such as endolymphatic sac decompression) can be offered.

Alternatively, IT gentamicin may be offered as a minimally invasive vestibular-ablative therapy to patients with no serviceable hearing, significant surgical risk, or failed endolymphatic sac decompression. Gentamicin is preferred over other amino-glycosides owing to its higher affinity for vestibular hair cells than cochlear hair cells, theoretically reducing the risk of hearing loss. There is a wide literature base in IT gentamicin therapy, but there is no consensus on optimal dosing protocol.[20]

If IT gentamicin fails, then more invasive surgical options may be offered, such as vestibular nerve section or total labyrinthectomy.

Before beginning IT perfusion, a baseline audiogram and videonystagmograpghy is strongly recommended.

Steroids: Indications and Dosing Protocol

Intratympanic steroid perfusions for intractable Meniere's disease have been indicated for patients who have failed 6 months of conservative medical treatment.[21] The literature has shown mixed results for vertigo control, hearing loss, aural fullness, and tinnitus.[22] One randomized, placebo-controlled trial reported significant symptom improvement using a DX solution of 4 mg/mL injected once daily for 4 days followed by a period of observation.[23]

The frequency and dosage of IT steroid injections for Meniere's disease remains physician dependent. We perform weekly IT steroid perfusion of MP on a weekly basis for a maximum of 4 injections. The injection technique is the same as described for sudden sensorineural hearing loss.

Vestibulotoxic Drugs: Indications and Dosing Protocol

Dosing protocols for vestibulotoxic drugs can be characterized as "low-dose fixed" and "titration." In low-dose fixed protocols, a set number of injections are performed over the course of days to weeks. Titration protocols involve an initial injection, followed by additional injections over weeks to months until a stopping point is reached. Some studies report better vertigo control, less tinnitus, and better quality of life with titration protocols, although the evidence is not definitive.[20] The injection is performed in a similar manner to the methods above. Some protocols involve aspirating the gentamicin out of the middle ear at the end of the dwell time and some administer gentamicin via a pressure equalizer tube.[6] We perform one IT injection of 0.5 mL of gentamicin 40 mg/dL. If there are persistent symptoms after 1 month, we administer another injection.

SUMMARY

Recent advancements in otology have expanded the practice toward more minimally invasive treatments. Endoscopy allows greater visualization and access to portions of the tympanic membrane and middle ear cavity. Intratympanic therapy offers more non-surgical options. All of these implementations allow the surgeon to manage more patients in the office rather than the operating room, potentially avoiding risks, improving outcomes, and decreasing cost.

SUPPLEMENTARY DATA

Supplementary data related to this article can be found online at https://doi.org/10.1016/j.otc.2019.02.004.

REFERENCES

1. Sade J, Avraham S, Brown M. Atelectasis, retraction pockets and cholesteatoma. Acta Otolaryngol 1981;92(5–6):501–12.
2. Tos M, Poulsen G. Attic retractions following secretory otitis. Acta Otolaryngol 1980;89(5–6):479–86.
3. Yung M, Tono T, Olszewska E, et al. EAONO/JOS Joint Consensus Statements on the definitions, classification and staging of middle ear cholesteatoma. J Int Adv Otol 2017;13(1):1–8.
4. Poe DS, Rebeiz EE, Pankratov MM. Evaluation of perilymphatic fistulas by middle ear endoscopy. Am J Otol 1992;13(6):529–33.
5. Kakehata S. Transtympanic endoscopy for diagnosis of middle ear pathology. Otolaryngol Clin North Am 2013;46(2):227–32.

6. Silverstein H, Rowan PT, Olds MJ, et al. Inner ear perfusion and the role of round window patency. Am J Otol 1997;18(5):586–9.

7. Gun T, Sozen T, Boztepe OF, et al. Influence of size and site of perforation on fat graft myringoplasty. Auris Nasus Larynx 2014;41(6):507–12.

8. Saliba I, Woods O. Hyaluronic acid fat graft myringoplasty: a minimally invasive technique. Laryngoscope 2011;121(2):375–80.

9. D'Eredita R. Porcine small intestinal submucosa (SIS) myringoplasty in children: a randomized controlled study. Int J Pediatr Otorhinolaryngol 2015;79(7):1085–9.

10. James AL. Endoscope or microscope-guided pediatric tympanoplasty? Comparison of grafting technique and outcome. Laryngoscope 2017;127(11):2659–64.

11. Alper CM, Luntz M, Takahashi H, et al. Panel 2: anatomy (Eustachian tube, middle ear, and mastoid-anatomy, physiology, pathophysiology, and pathogenesis). Otolaryngol Head Neck Surg 2017;156(4_suppl):S22–40.

12. Pelikan Z. Role of nasal allergy in chronic secretory otitis media. Curr Allergy Asthma Rep 2009;9(2):107–13.

13. Salt AN, Plontke SK. Principles of local drug delivery to the inner ear. Audiol Neurootol 2009;14(6):350–60.

14. Stachler RJ, Chandrasekhar SS, Archer SM, et al. Clinical practice guideline: sudden hearing loss. Otolaryngol Head Neck Surg 2012;146(3 Suppl):S1–35.

15. Rauch SD, Halpin CF, Antonelli PJ, et al. Oral vs intratympanic corticosteroid therapy for idiopathic sudden sensorineural hearing loss: a randomized trial. JAMA 2011;305(20):2071–9.

16. Wilson WR, Byl FM, Laird N. The efficacy of steroids in the treatment of idiopathic sudden hearing loss. A double-blind clinical study. Arch Otolaryngol 1980; 106(12):772–6.

17. Han X, Yin X, Du X, et al. Combined intratympanic and systemic use of steroids as a first-line treatment for sudden sensorineural hearing loss: a meta-analysis of randomized, controlled trials. Otol Neurotol 2017;38(4):487–95.

18. Parnes LS, Sun AH, Freeman DJ. Corticosteroid pharmacokinetics in the inner ear fluids: an animal study followed by clinical application. Laryngoscope 1999;109(7 Pt 2):1–17.

19. Demirhan H, Gökduman AR, Hamit B, et al. Contribution of intratympanic steroids in the primary treatment of sudden hearing loss. Acta Otolaryngol 2018;138(7): 648–51.

20. Schoo DP, Tan GX, Ehrenburg MR, et al. Intratympanic (IT) therapies for Meniere's disease: some consensus among the confusion. Curr Otorhinolaryngol Rep 2017; 5(2):132–41.

21. Clyde JW, Oberman BS, Isildak H. Current management practices in Meniere's disease. Otol Neurotol 2017;38(6):e159–67.

22. Lavigne P, Lavigne F, Saliba I. Intratympanic corticosteroids injections: a systematic review of literature. Eur Arch Otorhinolaryngol 2016;273(9):2271–8.

23. Garduno-Anaya MA, Couthino De Toledo H, Hinojosa-Gonzalez R, et al. Dexamethasone inner ear perfusion by intratympanic injection in unilateral Meniere's disease: a two-year prospective, placebo-controlled, double-blind, randomized trial. Otolaryngol Head Neck Surg 2005;133(2):285–94.

In-Office Balloon Dilation of the Eustachian Tube under Local Anesthesia

Marc Dean, MD[a],*, Melissa A. Pynnonen, MD, MSc[b]

KEYWORDS

• Balloon dilation • Eustachian tube • Local anesthesia • In-office procedure

KEY POINTS

• Ideal patients have had symptoms for longer than 12 weeks and have type B or C tympanograms despite maximal medical therapy.
• Using an angled endoscope to directly visualize the ET orifice throughout the procedure is critical to a successful outcome.
• Anesthetizing the mechanoreceptors in both the tympanic membrane and the nasopharynx maximize patient comfort during the procedure.

 Video content accompanies this article at http://www.oto.theclinics.com.

HISTORY OF EUSTACHIAN TUBE ANATOMY AND FUNCTION

The Eustachian tube (ET) was first mentioned by Aristotle in the fourth century BC but it is named after Bartolomeus Eustachius who described its anatomy in 1562.[1] At that time the function of the ET was believed to be an avenue for hearing or respiration. It was not until 1683 when Duverney proposed that the ET served as the channel through which the air of the middle ear was renewed that the actual function of the ET was first postulated. Finally, with the advent of fiberoptic endoscopy in the late 20th century the dynamic nature of the ET was understood.[2]

EUSTACHIAN TUBE FUNCTION

We now understand that the ET regulates middle ear pressure with respect to atmosphere pressure, facilitates clearance of middle ear secretions, and protects the middle ear from

Disclosure Statement: Dr. Dean is a consultant for Acclarent Inc., Biosense Webster, Bioinspire, Airnex, and Immertec, and hope equity or stock options in BioInspire; Immertec; and This American Doc (TAD).
^a Vitruvio Institute for Medical Advancement, Texas Tech University Health Science Center, Lubbock, TX, USA; ^b Otolaryngology, West Ann Arbor Health Center, University of Michigan, 380 Parkland Plaza, Ann Arbor, MI 48103-6021, USA
* Corresponding author. 901 Hemphill Street, Fort Worth, TX 76104.
E-mail address: Marc.Dean@gmail.com

Otolaryngol Clin N Am 52 (2019) 509–520
https://doi.org/10.1016/j.otc.2019.02.005
0030-6665/19/© 2019 The Authors. Published by Elsevier Inc. This is an open access article under the CC BY-NC-ND license (http://creativecommons.org/licenses/by-nc-nd/4.0/).

Abbreviations/acronyms	
ATM	Atmospheric pressure
BDET	Balloon dilation of the eustachian tube
CT	Computerized tomography
ECOG	Electrocochleography
ET	Eustachian tube
ETD	Eustachian tube dysfunction
ETDQ-7	Eustachian Tube Dysfunction Questionnaire-7
IAC	Internal auditory canal
LPR	Laryngopharyngeal reflux
TM	Tympanic membrane
VEMP	Vestibular evoked myogenic potential

sound and accumulation of nasopharyngeal secretions.[3] This is due to a dynamic valve-like region created by the insertion of the tensor veli palatine muscle located 12 to 20 mm distal to the nasopharyngeal orifice. The tensor veli palatine contracts, initiating a coordinated sequence in concert with the other peri-tubal muscles, which opens the ET.

THREE CATEGORIES OF EUSTACHIAN TUBE DYSFUNCTION

Eustachian tube dysfunction (ETD) refers to inadequate function of the ET and is defined in 3 categories: dilatory, patulous, and barometric challenge. Dilatory ETD refers to the inability of the valve to appropriately open the ET, leading to negative pressure in the middle ear.[4] Patulous ETD is at the other end of the spectrum and refers to the inability of the ET to appropriately close causing autophony.[3] The third category, barometric challenge ETD results from the inability of the ET to regulate acute pressure changes, for example, when flying or diving. Dilatory ETD is the form most amenable to balloon treatment, and dilatory ETD is the focus of the remainder of this article.

Dilatory Eustachian Tube Dysfunction

Typical dilatory ETD is characterized by signs and symptoms of negative pressure in the middle ear. Common symptoms include aural fullness with hearing loss or tinnitus. When severe, patients may experience otalgia and may develop serous otitis media and complications such as atelectasis, retraction pockets, or even cholesteatoma.[2,5] Work by Poe and colleagues,[6] has shown that the most common cause of dilatory ETD is mucosal inflammation within the cartilaginous ET, often because of allergic rhinitis, chronic rhinosinusitis, laryngopharyngeal reflux (LPR), or exposure to tobacco smoke.

Dilatory ETD affects 30% to 80% of people at some point during childhood.[7] Despite the maturation of the ET and the management of underlying causes, ETD continues to plague approximately 1% of the population throughout their adult lives.[3]

AURAL FULLNESS WORK UP

Patients with ETD typically present with aural fullness or hearing loss. Common causes of ETD include allergic rhinitis, chronic rhinosinusitis LPR, and barometric pressure changes. Eustachian tube dysfunction is often multi-factorial and it is important that all contributing factors are identified. It is also essential to recognize conditions that mimic ETD including temporal mandibular joint disorders, nasopharyngeal mass, cochlear hydrops, and superior canal dehiscence. Physicians can differentiate among the various forms of ETD and other common causes of aural fullness with a history, physical examination, and directed testing as depicted in the flowchart in **Fig. 1**.

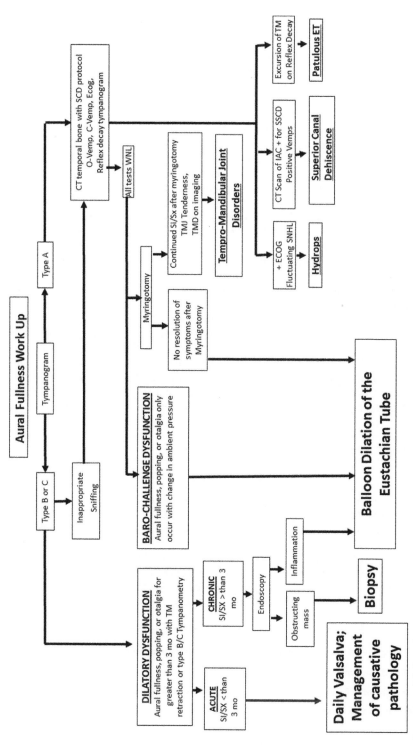

Fig. 1. Aural fullness work up.

Type A Tympanogram

Testing for all patients with aural fullness begins with audiogram and tympanometry. If the patient has a type A tympanogram additional testing is necessary. Tympanic reflex testing should be obtained to look for decay caused by excessive excursion of the tympanic membrane (TM), suggesting patulous ETD. A history of sensitivity or vertigo when exposed to loud sounds suggests superior canal dehiscence syndrome. This can be corroborated with a non-contrast computerized tomography (CT) scan of the temporal bones and internal auditory canals (IACs) with 0.5-mm cuts reformatted in the plane parallel and perpendicular to the superior semicircular canal demonstrating dehiscence of the superior semicircular canal,[8] and vestibular evoked myogenic potentials (VEMPS) that show abnormally low thresholds and enlarged amplitudes.[9] Electrocochleography (ECOG) testing should be considered if the aural fullness is also accompanied by fluctuating hearing loss to rule out cochlear hydrops (**Box 1**).

If the diagnostic work up is normal or inconsistent with the patient's symptoms, it is often useful to perform a myringotomy. Myringotomy improves middle ear ventilation. If the symptoms resolve after the myringotomy it is likely the patients symptoms will resolve after balloon dilation of the Eustachian tube (BDET), which also improves ventilation of the middle ear. However, if the symptoms persist following myringotomy it is recommended to evaluate for a temporal mandibular joint disorder, as it can cause aural fullness.[3]

Finally, patients with type A tympanograms, normal tympanic reflex decay, normal CT cervical VEMPS, and ocular VEMPS ECOG and without symptom resolution following myringotomy may have barometric challenge ETD. This is less common than dilatory ETD and is defined as aural fullness and pain when presented with a barometric challenge. These patients are more difficult to diagnose because their symptoms are transient and only occur with barometric pressure changes. Balloon dilation of the Eustachian tube is very effective in patients with barometric challenge ETD.

Type B or C Tympanogram

A type B or C tympanogram suggests dilatory ETD. Further testing may be unnecessary, although a temporal bone CT scan should be considered in the setting of an atypical history or unclear pathology. A CT scan can be beneficial also in understanding the relation between the internal carotid artery and the ET, as well as identifying potential obstructing pathology such as cartilaginous anomalies or tumors.[10]

Otoscopy in patients with dilatory ETD may reveal TM retraction or effusion. It is important to remember that while retraction pockets in the posterior superior quadrant or attic may have originated from ETD, they may persist or progress because of unrelated inflammatory mechanisms, despite the resolution of ETD.

Box 1
Work up patients with suspected ETD and a type A tympanogram

- Reflex decay tympanogram
- Non-contrast CT scan of the temporal bones and IACs "superior canal dehiscence protocol"
- Cervical VEMPS and ocular VEMPS
- ECOG

Nasal endoscopy is used to evaluate for inflammatory or neoplastic disease. The ET orifice is located just posterior to the inferior turbinate. To optimize the view of the ET orifice during opening and closing, a flexible endoscope should be brought to the tubal orifice and directed 45° laterally and superiorly relative to the nasal floor. This can be accomplished from the ipsilateral or contralateral nasal cavity.[6] The most common findings seen in dilatory ETD include mucosal inflammation, hypertrophy, excessive mucus, hyperemia, and cobble-stoning.[3]

Dilatory ETD must be differentiated from patulous ETD. A patient with dilatory ETD typically has a type B or C tympanogram. In contrast, a patient with patulous ETD will have a type A tympanogram, positive reflex decay, and will report autophony and fullness that worsens with activity. Atelectasis, non-fixed TM retraction, or middle ear effusion suggest dilatory ETD, whereas medial and lateral excursions of the TM with ipsilateral nasal breathing indicate patulous ETD. If patulous ETD is suspected, having the patient exercise for several minutes before otoscopy may provoke symptoms and visible TM movement with respiration.[11]

Patients with aural fullness should complete a Eustachian Tube Dysfunction Questionnaire-7 (ETDQ-7) survey to assess symptom burden. The ETDQ-7 is a symptom scale developed by McCoul and colleagues.[12] Patients are surveyed about pressure, ear pain, a feeling of clogged or muffled hearing, ear symptoms during sinusitis or common cold, crackling sounds or tinnitus in one or both ears over the last month. Patients respond with a number from 1 to 7 (no problem to severe problem).

TREATMENT OF DILATORY EUSTACHIAN TUBE DYSFUNCTION

Medical treatment of ETD consisting of routinely performing a Valsalva maneuver and either 4 weeks of nasal steroids or 1 week of oral steroids should be performed before considering BDET. Although it has not been demonstrated to significantly alter the course of refractory ETD, it does help establish candidacy for BDET.[13]

Kujawaski ushered in the modern era of ET surgery in 1997 by describing the first Eustachian tuboplasty. He approached the ET both transorally and transnasally to obliterate mucosa and cartilage from the posterior cushion using a laser.[1] Ten years later, Metson described an exclusively transnasal approach that used a powered shaver such as is commonly used in endoscopic sinus surgery.[14]

In 2009, Ockermann and colleagues described the first use of a noncompliant balloon to treat dilatory ETD. In 2010, Ockermann and colleagues[15] published their study exploring the use of sinus balloons as a device to treat dilatory ETD. One of the advantages of BDET over other treatments for ETD is that it directly targets the cause of dilatory ETD at both the mucosal and submucosal level. Kivekäs and colleagues[16] demonstrated histologic evidence that the balloon causes both shear and crush injury of the epithelium, but spares the basal layer, allowing for rapid healing. In addition, the balloon crushes lymphocytes and lymphoid follicles within the submucosa leading to the formation of a fibrous scar. This combination significantly reduces the overall inflammatory burden and may provide lasting clinical improvement in ET dilatory function and middle ear ventilation.

Over the last 10 years BDET has been demonstrated to be efficacious. Multiple studies have demonstrated symptomatic as well as objective clinical improvement in patients undergoing BDET for ETD.[3,13,17] Balloon dilation of the Eustachian tube has success rates ranging from 64% to 97% and a complication rate of approximately 2%.[17] In a recent multi-institutional randomized trial of patients with chronic ETD, Poe and colleagues[13] demonstrated that, at 6-week follow-up, treated compared with untreated patients experienced normalization of tympanograms (51.8% versus 13.9%)

and ETDQ-7 scores (56.2% versus 8.5%). Balloon dilation of the Eustachian tube has emerged as the surgical treatment of choice for dilatory ETD, and there is growing interest in performing this procedure in the office.

As with any new procedure, determining who will benefit, can be challenging. A recent randomized controlled trial demonstrated the effectiveness of BDET in patients with ETD, as defined by aural fullness greater than 12 weeks in combination with a type B or C tympanogram, along with a positive ETDQ-7 score greater than 14 despite either using nasal steroids for at least 4 weeks or oral steroids for 1 week (**Box 2**).[13]

Physicians should be cautious when considering in-office BDET for patients with barometric-induced ETD. Balloon dilation of the Eustachian tube changes the barometric pressure in the middle ear, which may trigger pain or vertigo. These symptoms can be mitigated by using a vestibular suppressant such as diazepam, anesthetizing the TM, which blunts the isobarometric reflex arc, and inflating the balloon slowly, at a rate of 1 atmospheric pressure (ATM) per second.

Successful BDET improves ET function and normalizes middle ear pressure. Following the procedure, most patients can Valsalva immediately and many report benefit within a few days. This can be objectively followed by tympanograms, and clinically followed with ETDQ-7 scores. The tympanograms and ETDQ-7 scores usually normalize within 6 weeks and these results have been shown durable over time.[13,17]

PRE-TREATMENT PLANNING

Before considering BDET under local anesthesia, nasopharyngoscopy should be performed to evaluate the patient for any anatomic challenges that may complicate the procedure or require additional surgical intervention for access. Special attention should be given to the nasal airway, looking for a nasal obstruction, such as septal deviations or spurs, extension of the inferior turbinate into the nasal airway, as well as lateral adenoid hypertrophy. If any of these findings are present it may make the procedure challenging and the physician may prefer to perform BDET as well as any additional indicated procedure in a more controlled environment.

ANESTHETIC CONSIDERATIONS

Adequate anesthesia is critical to the success of in-office BDET. There are 3 specific considerations. First, the transnasal approach to the nasopharynx requires good topical anesthesia for the nasal cavity. Second, mechanical receptors of the TM, promontory, and nasopharynx create a neuronal reflex arc that regulates pressure in the middle ear. These receptors are uniquely sensitive to the barometric changes that will be induced during the procedure.[18] Third, BDET can induce pressure changes in the middle ear possibly inducing vertigo. Thus, anesthesia must be provided with attention to all 3 of these concerns.[19]

Box 2
Ideal candidate for BDET

- Aural fullness greater than 12 weeks
- Type B or C tympanogram
- ETDQ-7 score greater than 14
- Failed medical management including Valsalva and either 4 weeks of nasal steroids or 1 week of oral steroids

PATIENT POSITIONING AND ANESTHETIC ADMINISTRATION

To minimize discomfort as well as limit vertigo, patients should be premedicated with a vestibular suppressant such as 10 mg of diazepam 90 minutes before the procedure. On arrival to the office the patient should be evaluated and if necessary another 10 mg of diazepam along with 5 mg of hydrocodone can be administered.

The patient should then be positioned at 45° angle in either an examination room chair or procedure table. Oxymetazoline should be sprayed into each nostril, 5 drops 7% tetracaine/7% lidocaine compounded into an otic solution should be placed onto the ipsilateral TM via the external auditory canal, and 2 cottonoids soaked in 2% tetracaine should be placed along the nasal floor bilaterally and left to sit for approximately 10 minutes. The cottonoids should then be removed and approximately 0.5 mL of compounded 7% tetracaine/7% lidocaine cream should be applied to the ET orifice via a low profile cannula such as the Weiss catheter (Grace Medical, Memphis, TN, USA). This, in combination with the topical anesthetic drops placed on the TM earlier, disrupt the isobarometric reflex arc. The tetracaine-soaked cottonoids should then be replaced and allowed to sit for another 10 to 15 minutes (**Box 3**). The cottonoids can then be removed and the procedure initiated.

EQUIPMENT AND SUPPLIES

The endoscope runs parallel to the dilation device throughout most of the procedure, so it is recommended that a monitor and endoscopic camera be used along with an angled endoscope to maximize visualization.

In addition to using an angled endoscope, it is important to be aware of the endoscope's length before the procedure. Some of the shorter endoscopes can easily get caught on the dilation systems, preventing advancement of the balloon catheter in to the ET lumen.

It is also important to have suction available to evacuate any fluids that might obstruct the orifice or true lumen of the ET. The suction catheter can also function as a cannula to deliver the topical anesthesia to the lumen of the ET.

TECHNICAL DETAILS

Balloon dilation of the Eustachian tube should be performed with a 30° or 45° rigid endoscope to allow for direct visualization of the ET orifice as shown in Video 1. This direct view with an angled endoscope significantly reduces the risk for inadvertent tissue trauma and creation of false passages. Currently there are 2 dilation systems approved by the Federal Drug Administration for use under local anesthesia,

---

Box 3
Local anesthesia protocol

- 10 mg diazepam 90 minutes before the procedure
- 5 mg hydrocodone 30 minutes before the procedure
- 4 sprays of oxymetazoline to each nostril
- 5 drops compounded 7% tetracaine/7% lidocaine drops on TM
- 2% tetracaine-soaked cottonoids along the nasal floor bilaterally
- 0.5 mL 7% tetracaine/7% lidocaine cream in ET orifice
- Replace tetracaine-soaked cottonoids along the nasal floor

and although they both use a noncompliant balloon, the catheters themselves differ significantly (see Video 1).

The AERA Dilation System

The AERA Dilation system (Acclarent, Irvine CA, USA) uses a 55° angled guide to introduce a 6 × 16-mm noncompliant flexible balloon catheter into the nasopharyngeal orifice of the ET. Under direct visualization, the balloon catheter should be gently advanced superiorly, navigating the S-shaped curve in the ET until the catheter encounters resistance at the bony-cartilaginous isthmus. Once the balloon is fully inserted into the cartilaginous ET, the yellow mark indicates the end of the balloon and should be visible along the medial edge of the anterior cushion of the ET, ensuring the balloon is not inserted too deeply. The assistant then inflates the balloon at approximately 1 ATM per second until the pressure reaches 12 ATM. The balloon should then be held in the inflated position for 2 minutes then deflated and slowly retracted into the guide. The entire system is then withdrawn from the nose.[20]

The Xpress Dilation System

The Xpress Dilation system (Entellus, Plymouth MN, USA) rigid balloon catheter was originally designed for dilation of the sinus ostia, but has been adapted for BDET and is available in diameters of 5, 6, and 7 mm and lengths of 8, 18, and 20 mm, which slide along a reshapeable ridged rail. The manufacturer's instructions contain little information to inform the choice of balloon size. However, most of the data in the scientific literature have been generated with a 6 × 16-mm balloon. The distal end of the rail contains a 2-cm mark. At this location the rail should be bent approximately 45°. This bend will be a visual indicator of the depth of ET cannulation. Then, under direct visualization, the rigid rail is introduced into the ET orifice, and advanced until the angle of the rigid rail is even with the medial edge of the anterior cushion of the ET. The balloon is then advanced along the rail to its full length until the balloon cannot be advanced any further, indicating that the balloon has reached the tip of the rail. The assistant inflates the balloon approximately 1 ATM per second until it reaches 12 ATM. It is held into position for 2 minutes and then deflated. Because of the length of the cartilaginous ET (on average 24 mm long), the instructions for use recommend performing 2 dilations at staggered lengths based on device markings when using the 8 mm balloon to achieve the desired result. The balloon dilation system is then removed.[21]

TIPS AND SAFETY CONSIDERATIONS

Regardless of which balloon system is used, the technical tips listed in **Box 4** can make the procedure easier for the surgeon and more comfortable for the patient.

Box 4
Technical tips

- Gently retract the posterior cushion medially with the rail or guide, to allow for visualization of the ET lumen, providing guidance while advancing the balloon.
- Avoid removing the balloon while inflated, as the resultant negative pressure can cause significant discomfort
- Slow dilation at 1 ATM per second minimizes the risk of triggering the isobarrometric arc, allowing for a more comfortable procedure

---

Balloon dilation of the Eustachian tube is a relatively safe procedure; however, because of the anatomic location of the ET, as well as its role in regulating middle ear pressure, there are several safety considerations that should be kept in mind when performing this procedure in the office.

Sudden pressure changes within the middle ear can precipitate vertigo. In addition to premedication with a vestibular suppressant such as diazepam, the risk of vertigo can be mitigated by ensuring that the central lumen of the balloon catheter is free of guidewires and other obstructions to allow for release of back pressure during dilation. Todt and colleagues[22] demonstrated that middle ear pressure during BDET depends on the speed of inflation and maximum inflation pressure. Middle ear pressure during dilation averages approximately 71 daPa, and while this is not enough to rupture the round window or healthy TM, it can cause significant discomfort. Connecting the ventilation ports to suction should also be avoided as the resultant negative pressure generated in the middle ear can be uncomfortable.

POTENTIAL COMPLICATIONS

The overall safety profile of the procedure is quite good; however, minor tears of the mucosal lumen, epistaxis, exacerbation of tinnitus, temporary deafness or vertigo, and subcutaneous emphysema and patulous ETD have been reported after BDET.[3]

Temporary deafness and vertigo may occur related to the topical anesthetic. When applying topical anesthesia within the ET it important to use a cream or ointment rather than a gel, which has a potential to liquefy at body temperature and has a risk of being absorbed into the inner ear via the round window and cause symptoms. For this reason, it is also important to evaluate the TM before placing the medication in the external ear canal to rule out any perforations or patent pressure equalization tubes.

The risk of a false passage can be decreased by using an angled endoscope to directly visualize the ET lumen, especially when navigating the balloon through the S-shaped curve of the ET. Natural tissue planes provide little resistance to penetration by either the balloon catheter or shapeable rail depending on the system used. Without direction visualization, one may be unaware of being in a false passage. It is important to recognize this when it occurs and cannulate the true lumen before dilating, not only to avoid damaging surrounding soft tissue, but also to ensure the balloon has an opportunity to come in contact with the respiratory epithelium during inflation. When a false passage does occur, it is important to counsel the patient not to Valsalva and sneeze with their mouth open to minimize the risk of subcutaneous emphysema.

RECOVERY

Patients usually recover easily. Their post-treatment symptoms are most often characterized by aural fullness due to ET trauma produced by the procedure. Nausea, nasal congestion, epistasis, vertigo, ear and neck pain, headache, and sore throat occasionally occur and usually resolve quickly.

POST-OPERATIVE INSTRUCTIONS

Patients should continue the use of nasal steroids, as well as gently performing the Valsalva maneuver every hour while awake. If there is any concern for a false passage or mucosal tear it is recommended to wait at least a week before attempting the Valsalva maneuver, sneeze with their mouth open, refrain from flying, lifting heavy objects, or forcefully blowing their nose for 2 weeks after the procedure to minimize the risk of subcutaneous emphysema. It also beneficial to keep the head elevated for the first 48 to 72 hours to reduce swelling within the ET. Over-the-counter analgesics such as acetaminophen or non-steroidal anti-inflammatory drugs are usually sufficient to cover any post-operative pain.

OUTCOMES

Most studies in the literature describe BDET performed under general anesthesia. However, in one of the first studies looking at the effectiveness of BDET, Catalano and colleagues[23] retrospectively reviewed 100 cases BDET, of which 37% of the procedures were performed under local anesthesia in the office. The patients had an average follow-up of 26 weeks, 71% of patients experienced improvement in ear fullness and pressure and 87% reported persistent improvement. The average dilation time varied between 10 and 30 seconds, with a pressure of 6 to 8 ATM, and with some of the procedures having to be discontinued after 10 seconds because of pain. As the technique of BDET has evolved, it has become customary to dilate the ET for approximately 2 minutes with a pressure of 10 to 12 ATM.[24]

In a recent randomized controlled trial looking at clinical efficacy, BDET showed significant improvement in ETDQ-7 scores at 6 weeks, and that improvement was maintained through 12 months. Importantly 72% of the procedures were performed under local anesthesia with no complications, and all patients tolerated the procedure.[25]

CODING, BILLING, AND REIMBURSEMENT

Balloon dilation of the Eustachian tube is a relatively new procedure and currently lacks a specific current procedural terminology code for the procedure. The AMA recommends the use of the middle ear unlisted code, 69799. This code lacks specific reimbursement recommendations based on the site of service designations, and, as a result, it is difficult to receive sufficient reimbursement from third-party payers to cover the cost of the devices required to perform this procedure in the office. However, it has been the author's experience that most patients are willing to cover the cost of the procedure in exchange for the benefits of undergoing this procedure in the office setting.

SUMMARY

Dilatory ETD has long posed significant diagnostic and treatment challenges to the clinician. Recent advances in technology have led to a better understanding of the dynamic function of the ET, allowing for more effective treatment options. Balloon dilation of the Eustachian tube has emerged as a promising treatment of dilatory ETD. With the right patient selection, operative technique, and anesthesia protocol, BDET can easily be performed in an office setting under local anesthesia, significantly reducing cost and minimizing the risk of general anesthesia.

SUPPLEMENTARY DATA

Supplementary data related to this article can be found online at https://doi.org/10.1016/j.otc.2019.02.005.

REFERENCES

1. McCoul ED, Lucente FE, Anand VK. Evolution of Eustachian tube surgery. Laryngoscope 2011;121:661–6.

2. Bluestone CD. Introduction. In: Bluestone MB, editor. Eustachian tube: structure, function, role in otitis media. New York: B C Decker; 2005. p. 1–9.
3. Adil E, Poe D. What is the full range of medical and surgical treatments available for patients with Eustachian tube dysfunction? Curr Opin Otolaryngol Head Neck Surg 2014;22:8–15.
4. Seibert JW, Danner CJ. Eustachian tube function and the middle ear. Otolaryngol Clin North Am 2006;39:122118.
5. Schilder AGM, Bhutta MF, Butler CC, et al. Eustachian tube dysfunction: consensus statement on definition, types, clinical presentation and diagnosis. Clin Otolaryngol 2015;40:407–11.
6. Poe DS, Pyykko I, Valtonen H, et al. Analysis of Eustachian tube function by video endoscopy. Am J Otol 2000;21:602–7.
7. Browning GG, Gatehouse S. The prevalence of middle ear disease in the adult British population. Clin Otolaryngol 1992;17:317–21.
8. Sparacia G, Iaia A. Diagnostic performance of reformatted isotropic thin-section helical CT images in the detection of superior semicircular canal dehiscence. Neuroradiol J 2017;30(3):216–21.
9. Brantberg K, Bergenius J, Tribukait A. Vestibular-evoked myogenic potentials in patients with dehiscence of the superior semicircular canal. Acta Otolaryngol 1999;119(6):633–40.
10. Abdel-Aziz T, Schroder S, Lehmann M, et al. Computed tomography before balloon Eustachian tuboplasty - a true necessity? Otol Neurotol 2014;35:635–8.
11. Poe DS. Diagnosis and management of the patulous Eustachian tube. Otol Neurotol 2007;28:668–77.
12. McCoul ED, Anand VK, Christos PJ. Validating the clinical assessment of Eustachian tube dysfunction: the Eustachian Tube Dysfunction Questionnaire (ETDQ-7). Laryngoscope 2012;122(5):1137–41.
13. Poe D, Anand V, Dean M, et al. Balloon dilation of the Eustachian tube for dilatory dysfunction: a randomized controlled trial. Laryngoscope 2018;128(5):1200–6.
14. Metson R, Pletcher SD, Poe DS. Microdebrider Eustachian tuboplasty: a preliminary report. Otolaryngol Head Neck Surg 2007;136:422–7.
15. Ockermann T, Reinke U, Upile T, et al. Balloon dilation Eustachian tuboplasty: a clinical study. Laryngoscope 2010;120(7):1411–6.
16. Kivekäs I, Chao WC, Faquin W, et al. Histopathology of balloon-dilation Eustachian tuboplasty. Laryngoscope 2015;125:436–41.
17. Huisman JML, Verdam FJ, Stegeman I, et al. Treatment of Eustachian tube dysfunction with balloon dilation a systematic review. Laryngoscope 2018; 128(1):237–47.
18. Songu M, Aslan A, Unlu HH, et al. Neural control of Eustachian tube function. Laryngoscope 2009;119:1198–202.
19. Salburgo F, Garcia S, Lagier A, et al. Histological identification of nasopharyngeal mechanoreceptors. Eur Arch Otorhinolaryngol 2016;273(12):4127–33.
20. ACCLARENT AERA Eustachian tube balloon dilation system instructions for use. Irvine (CA): Acclarent, INC; 2018. IFU005146 Rev E.
21. XprESS ENT dilation system instructions for use. Plymouth (MN): Entellus Medical Inc.; 2017. IFU003563-002.
22. Todt I, Abdel-Aziz T, Mittmann P, et al. Measurement of middle ear pressure changes during balloon Eustachian tuboplasty: a pilot study. Acta Otolaryngol 2017;137(5):471–5.
23. Catalano PJ, Jonnalagadda S, Yu VM. Balloon catheter dilation of Eustachian tube: a preliminary study. Otol Neurotol 2012;33:1549–52.

24. Luukkainen V, Kivekas I, Hammaren-Malmi S, et al. Balloon Eustachian tuboplasty under local anesthesia: is it feasible? Laryngoscope 2017;127:1021–5.

25. Meyer TA, O'Malley EM, Schlosser RJ, et al. A randomized controlled trial of balloon dilation as a treatment for persistent Eustachian tube dysfunction with 1-year follow-up. Otol Neurotol 2018;39(7):894–902.

In-Office Laryngology Injections

Gregory R. Dion, MD, MS*, Skyler W. Nielsen, DO

KEYWORDS

- Dysphonia • Vocal cord paralysis • Vocal fold lesion • Cough
- Spasmodic dysphonia

KEY POINTS

- In-office vocal fold augmentation can treat glottic insufficiency, vocal fold paresis/paralysis, and vocal fold atrophy using various injectable materials.
- Depending on surgeon comfort, available equipment, and patient anatomy/comfort, the per-oral, thyrohyoid, cricothyroid, transthyroid cartilage, and transnasal are all approaches for in-office injection augmentation.
- Adductor, abductor, and mixed types of spasmodic dysphonia are treated with in-office laryngeal botulinum toxin injections under EMG guidance, visual techniques, or into the false vocal folds.
- In-office vocal fold steroid injections are a useful adjunct treatment and demonstrate promising results for treating vocal fold scar or benign vocal fold lesions.
- Carefully assessed neurogenic cough may benefit from a variety of different forms of in-office laryngeal injections to include botulinum toxin, steroids, superior laryngeal nerve blocks, and augmentation.

INTRODUCTION

Advances in distal chip videolaryngoscopy equipment allows in-office laryngeal injections to provide a viable alternative to microdirect laryngoscopy under general anesthesia in many scenarios. Benefits of in-office laryngeal injections include decreased cost, avoiding general anesthesia, and the ability to titrate material delivered using patient feedback to optimize voice outcomes.[1] For example, an estimated $8250 is potentially saved by performing in-office injection laryngoplasty compared with the

Disclosure Statement: The views expressed in this manuscript are those of the authors and do not reflect the official policy or position of the Department of the Army, Department of the Air Force, Department of Defense, or the US Government.
Department of Otolaryngology–Head and Neck Surgery, Brooke Army Medical Center, 3551 Roger Brooke Drive, JBSA Fort Sam Houston, San Antonio, TX 78234, USA
* Corresponding author. Dental and Craniofacial Trauma Research Department, U.S. Army Institute of Surgical Research, 3698 Chambers Pass, Bldg 3611, JBSA Fort Sam Houston, San Antonio, TX 78234-7313, USA
E-mail address: gregory.r.dion.mil@mail.mil

Otolaryngol Clin N Am 52 (2019) 521–536
https://doi.org/10.1016/j.otc.2019.02.006
0030-6665/19/Published by Elsevier Inc.

Abbreviations/acronyms	
ABSD	Abductor spasmodic dysphonia
ADSD	Adductor spasmodic dysphonia
BTX	Botulinum toxin
SD	Spasmodic dysphonia
VFSI	Vocal fold steroid injection

operating room.[1] Research suggests equipment acquisition costs for in-office procedures offset over time with increased office-based procedures.[2] Also, whereas heart rate variability has been documented with in-office procedures, they are largely safe.[3] Common office injections covered in this article include:

- Injection laryngoplasty for vocal fold paralysis, paresis, and/or atrophy
- Laryngeal botulinum toxin injections for spasmodic dysphonia
- Subepithelial vocal fold steroid injections
- Steroid, botulinum toxin, and/or augmentation for neurogenic cough

INJECTION LARYNGOPLASTY
Introduction

Symptoms of glottic insufficiency include hoarseness, trouble swallowing, and aspiration.[4] Etiologies are true vocal fold paralysis or paresis, presbyphonia, or sulcus volcalis.[5] Voice therapy, injection laryngoplasty (in-office or operative), medialization laryngoplasty with Gore-Tex or a Silastic block, and laryngeal reinnervation procedures improve glottic insufficiency.[4] In-office injection augmentation is increasingly used, often as a temporizing measure while awaiting potential vocal fold motion recovery or as a trial procedure, increasing from 11% to 43% of augmentation procedures from 2003 to 2008.[6]

Vocal fold mobility impairment is best identified on flexible videolaryngoscopy, with flexible or rigid videostroboscopy providing additional detail in assessing vocal fold paresis, presbylarynges/vocal fold atrophy, and sulcus vocalis. In patients with mild glottic insufficiency, voice therapy is generally trialed first. If the glottal gap is large or vocal fold mobility impairment also affects swallow function, early medialization may prevent aspiration pneumonia, improve swallowing, and improve cough strength for mucus clearance.[7,8] A study by Rudolf and colleagues suggests that patients with a glottic gap more than 1 mm have 6 to 8 weeks of success with temporary augmentation, while those with 1 mm or less improved for at least 12 months. In general, a glottic gap 2 mm or less can effectively be treated with injection laryngoplasty, and those with 3 mm or more benefit from framework surgery.[5,9]

In-Office Augmentation Patient Selection

Patients with poor cognition and/or a depressed mental status are often unable to cooperate, as are children. In-office injection laryngoplasty is ideal for patients requiring temporary augmentation, for patients for whom general anesthesia poses a high risk, and for patients with challenging laryngoscopy exposure, such as those with spinal fusion or poor neck extension after radiation. Patients may remain on anticoagulation medications for injections in-office or under general anesthesia. There are also patients who are better served under general anesthesia. Considerations *against* in-office injection:

- Unfavorable anatomy (large tongue base, retroflexed epiglottis, elongated soft palate, anteriorly based cervical spine osteophytes, large septal deflection)[10]
- Previous intolerance to awake injection

- Uneven vocal fold levels (better served with medialization laryngoplasty and/or arytenoid adduction)[11]
- Need to palpate vocal folds

Injectables

Selection of a vocal fold injectable encompasses patient and provider goals, provider experience, and availability. Numerous materials have been used for vocal fold augmentation, from paraffin and Teflon to autologous fat and bovine collagen. More recently, carboxymethylcellulose, calcium hydroxyapatite, and hyaluronic acid have been the primary injectables because of their biocompatibility, availability, and ease of injection through fine gauge needles.

Calcium hydroxylapatite is popular because of its long (12–18 month) duration and safe side-effect profile. Care is required with calcium hydroxylapatite, as mucosal wave disruption can occur if injected too superficially, although it can safely be used by experienced providers in the office setting.[6,12,13] Shorter-acting material, such as gel foam or carboxymethylcellulose, may be desired, particularly if recovery of function is possible or for a trial injection before framework surgery or lipoaugmentation. After 9 to 12 months of paralysis, spontaneous recovery is rare.[5] **Table 1** outlines common injectables.

Approaches

Anesthesia and setup

The thyrohyoid, per-oral, transthyroid ala, cricothyroid, and the transnasal endoscopic approaches can be used. An approach is selected based on patient anatomy, surgeon comfort/experience, and available equipment/assistance; however, the surgeon should have at least 1 alternative approach in mind if she/he encounters challenges with the primary approach.[14] **Table 2** outlines advantages and disadvantages of each approach.

Regardless of the approach, the procedure begins with the patient situated in the sniffing position in the examination chair (**Fig. 1**). Unless performing a per-oral approach with a 70° rigid telescope, proper nasal anesthesia is essential. Typically, atomizer delivery of 4% lidocaine mixed in equal parts with oxymetazoline into the nasal cavity is adequate. Occasionally, lidocaine/oxymetazoline-soaked cotton pledget packing or 4% cocaine pledget packing for 5 to 10 minutes is required.

Per-oral approach

Per-oral augmentations use either a flexible laryngoscope or a rigid 70° angled telescope connected to a video tower. The rigid laryngoscope permits a single person technique when there is no available assistant, with the patient pulling their tongue forward. Oral anesthesia with 20% Benzocaine spray provides oropharyngeal anesthesia (note: methemoglobinemia is a rare but serious complication from 20% Benzocaine spray).[15] Topical laryngeal anesthesia using 4% lidocaine is dripped through an Abraham cannula per-orally, the side channel of a ported flexible laryngoscope, or trans-trachea via a needle.[10]

The patient maintains a sniffing position (neck flexed and head extended). A curved injector needle, such as the 27-gauge curved orotracheal injector device (Medtronic Xomed, Jackson, FL, USA) is used to perform the augmentation. Alternatively, commercially available injectables (Prolaryn Gel and Prolaryn Plus) include a 9-inch bendable needle for this purpose. The needle is fashioned in a gently rounded 90° angle for the patient's anatomy (**Fig. 2**). Once the needle is seen on the laryngoscope at the back of the oropharynx, the surgeon's hand is drawn

Table 1
Injection laryngoplasty materials

Material	Category	Duration	Location of Injection	Gauge Needle	Complications	Disadvantages
Bovine collagen (Zyplast, Phonagel)[17,19,44,45]	Xenograft	6 mo	Vibratory membrane, lateral to vocal ligament	27	Hypersensitivity reaction (3%), arthralgias, arthritis, fever, urticaria, generalized swelling	Need for skin testing 6 wk in advance
Allogenic collagen (Cymetra, Artecoll)[4,17,19,20,44-46]	Homograft	3–12 mo	Vibratory membrane, lateral to vocal ligament	22–27	Submucosal deposits, laryngeal abscess, foreign body reaction	Expensive
Autologous collagen[17]	Autograft	6 mo	Vibratory membrane, lateral to vocal ligament	27–30		Donor site morbidity, expensive
Gelfoam[17,45]	Synthetic	4–8 wk		18		Short duration
Autologous fat[5,17,19,44]	Autograft	Several years to permanent	Vibratory membrane, lateral to vocal ligament	18–22		Unpredictable absorption, donor site morbidity
Fascia[11,17,19,44]	Autograft	13 mo	Vibratory membrane, lateral to vocal ligament	18–22		Donor site morbidity, large bore needle required
Calcium hyrodxyapatite (Prolaryn Plus)[5,11,17,23,47]	Synthetic	18 mo to 5 y	Lateral to vocal ligament	26	Erythema, edema, foreign body giant cell reaction, hypervascularity, mucosal wave restriction, polyp	Absorption of gel carrier (10%–15% over-injection recommended)
Hyaluronic acid (Restylane)[5,11,48]	Xenograft	Variable, 4–24 mo		26	Inflammatory reaction, mucosal wave restriction	Not recommended for patients allergic to eggs
Carboxy-methycellulose (Prolaryn Gel)[11]	Synthetic	3 mo	Lateral to vocal ligament	27		

Table 2 Inject approaches		
Approaches	**Advantages**	**Disadvantages**
Per-oral	• Potential for single person • Visualization of needle penetrating vocal fold • No local injection	• Patient discomfort • Difficult if strong gag reflex • Material waste in long needle
Thyrohyoid	• Visualization of needle penetrating vocal fold	• Local skin injection required • Steep angle can be challenging
Cricothyroid	• Direct approach	• Local skin injection required • Greater potential for superficial injection • Inability to see needle penetrate vocal fold
Transthyroid ala	• Direct approach	• Local skin injection required • Difficult to perform in older adults due to calcified cartilage • Greater potential for superficial injection • Inability to see needle penetrate vocal fold
Transnasal endoscopic	• No local skin injection • Patient comfort • Visualization of needle penetrating vocal fold	• Difficult to assess medialization during injection • Material waste in long needle

superiorly, directing the needle tip lateral to the vocal ligament and slightly anterior-lateral to the vocal process. Over-injection is advisable due to aqueous carrier absorption.

Thyrohyoid approach
A dose of 1–2 mL of 1% lidocaine with 1:100,000 epinephrine is used as local anesthesia in the thyrohyoid space; an additional 0.5 mL of the local anesthetic can be

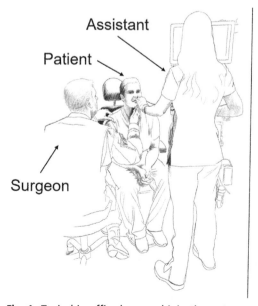
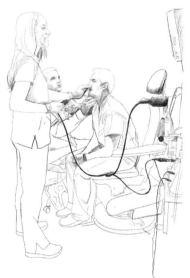

Assistant

Patient

Surgeon

Fig. 1. Typical in-office laryngeal injection setup.

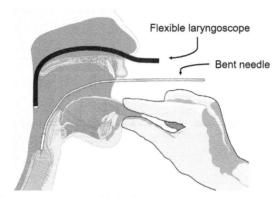

Flexible laryngoscope

Bent needle

Fig. 2. Sagittal illustration of per-oral injection.

placed in the pre-epiglottic space. Depending on equipment and surgeon comfort, topical laryngeal anesthesia can be accomplished with 4% lidocaine administered through the thyrohyoid needle, trans-trachea, or through the side channel of a ported flexible laryngoscope.

With an assistant maintaining laryngeal visualization on the video tower, a 25- or 27-gauge needle is inserted immediately superior to the thyroid notch and directed inferiorly, passing through the pre-epiglottic space. Careful back and forth motion of the needle indicates positioning on the monitor before entering the larynx. An additional small amount of 1% lidocaine with 1:100,000 epinephrine submucosally can decrease patient discomfort; if anesthetizing the larynx via this route, the needle is passed below the petiole just above the vocal folds, and 4% lidocaine is gently sprayed into the larynx as the patient holds an /i/ sound. For optimal augmentation, the needle should be oriented lateral to the vocal ligament and slightly anterior to the vocal process.[16] When needle orientation is inadequate, bending the needle anywhere from 45° to 90° near the hub and possibly again closer to the tip can aid in needle orientation, but may prevent optimal maneuverability for injection.[10]

Cricothyroid approach

Topical laryngeal anesthesia is generally not required with this approach, and local anesthesia is performed as discussed previously. A 23-, 25-, or 27-gauge needle is passed through the cricothyroid membrane under the thyroid ala approximately 5 to 7 mm from the midline. The needle is directed superiorly with the needle tip visualized on flexible laryngoscopy deep to the vocal fold epithelium. If the mucosa is being tented by the needle, the location is in the subepithelium, and the needle should be slightly withdrawn. A 30° to 45° needle bend superiorly can aid in achieving proper needle location.

Transthyroid ala approach

Local anesthesia is performed similar to the cricothyroid approach. A 25-gauge needle is positioned approximately 3 to 5 mm above the bottom of the thyroid ala, 6 to 12 mm from the midline, and oriented perpendicular to the thyroid cartilage. Once through the cartilage, the needle is gently moved back and forth to confirm positioning and the material is injected.[10] Because the needle must penetrate the thyroid cartilage, this approach is less favorable for older patients because of calcification.[17]

Transnasal endoscopic approach

With topical laryngeal anesthesia and positioning as described above, the surgeon maneuvers the laryngoscope while the assistant manages the ported laryngoscope's side channel. A flexible injection sheath is primed with injection material, and the flexible needle is passed through the sheathed working channel. Once past the distal tip of the laryngoscope, the needle is unsheathed and advanced into the proper location for injection. The flexible laryngoscope may need to be advanced slightly to overcome back pressure placed on the flexible needle.[18]

Post-operative Care

Generally, patients are advised to refrain from liquids and food for 1 hour after completion of the procedure to avoid inadvertent aspiration. Patients are observed in the office for approximately 20 minutes to ensure no respiratory distress or adverse reactions. There are no compelling data to warrant voice rest or steroids, and patients either resume normal phonation or are referred for voice therapy.

Outcomes

Patients should anticipate improved vocal volume, increased maximum phonation time, and improved stability after augmentation.[19] Technical success rate for in-office injections is approximately 97%, compared with 99% for injections in the operating room with comparable voice outcomes.[6] Failures in awake patients are usually attributed to patient discomfort, inadequate visualization, excessive secretions, or a prominent gag reflex. Vocal fold scars generally have a worse prognosis.[19]

Complications

Complications are uncommon, but include implant migration, suboptimal voice outcomes, vocal fold hematoma, vasovagal reaction, inability to complete procedure, revision surgery, and, rarely, airway compromise.[20] Studies showing no increased risk of hematoma in patients on anticoagulants.[7] When injected too superficially, materials, particularly calcium hydroxylapatite, may restrict mucosal wave requiring phonomicrosurgical correction.[21–23]

VOCAL FOLD STEROID INJECTIONS
Steroid Injections for Laryngeal Scars

Vocal fold scar (sulcus vocalis) originates after trauma, inflammation, and iatrogenically after surgery.[24] Corrective surgery is challenging with moderate improvements.[24] Vocal fold steroid injection (VFSI) of scars can improve mucosal wave and glottic closure.[24,25] Steroid injection volumes vary, and injections are commonly repeated after 6 to 12 weeks.[25]

Steroid Injections for Benign Vocal Fold Lesions

Benign vocal fold lesions encompass phonotraumatic lesions, polyps, Reinke edema, and intracordal cysts.[26] Voice therapy is the first line treatment, followed by phonomicrosurgery. Phonomicrosurgery for polyps and cysts remains the cornerstone of treatment; however, select lesions respond well to VFSI.[26,27] A meta-analysis found an 82% to 98% subjective improvement after VFSI for all benign vocal fold lesions combined, and an 89% to 100% partial response rate.[27] Adjuvant VFSI may also provide a faster resolution of the lesions.[28] **Table 3** outlines outcomes of VFSI for benign lesions.

Table 3
VFSI outcomes for benign vocal fold lesions

Study	Patients	Lesions	Follow-up Duration	Outcomes	Complications
Tateya et al,[49] 2003	44	Reinke edema	18 mo	32% complete resolution by endoscopy 64% partial resolution by endoscopy Subjective hoarseness improved/resolved in 98% Recurrence rate 30%	Not reported
Tateya et al,[50] 2004	28	Nodules	16 mo	63% complete resolution 37% partial resolution Subjective hoarseness improved/resolved in 96% Significant improvement in MPT (13.9 from 10.9) Recurrence rate 30%	Not reported
Mortensen and Woo,[25] 2006	34	Scars, polyps, nodules, cysts, granulomas	1 mo	82% reported subjective improvement Significant improvement in GRBAS Significant improvement in mucosal wave and amplitude on stroboscopy	Not reported
Hsu et al,[51] 2009	24	Polyps	15 mo	91% complete remission rate at 3 mo Significant improvement in GRBAS, VHI Significant improvement in MPT, Jitter, Shimmer, HNR 8.3% recurrence rate	Undefined occurrence of mucosal bleeding
Woo et al,[31] 2011	115	Nodules, polyps, cysts, Reinke edema	3 mo	35% complete remission 50% partial remission GRBAS, VHI significant improvement through 3 mo Jitter and Shimmer showed statistical improvement	1.6% hematoma Majority of patients white plaques

Study	N	Lesions treated	Follow-up	Outcomes	Complications
Wang et al,[29] 2013	30	Nodules, polyps	3 mo	97% of lesions resolved or improved on endoscopy; Significant improvement in VHI and GRB; Significant decrease in Jitter and Shimmer; Significant improvement in MPT (13.0 from 11.0)	10% hematoma rate
Wang et al,[26] 2015	126	Nodules, polyps, cysts	2 mo	80% reported subjective improvement; 80% had decreased lesion size; Significant improvement in VHI-10, VAS, and GRB scores; No significant improvement in MPT; 15%–20% complete resolution of nodule	27% hematoma; 4% white plaques; 0.7% temporary vocal fold atrophy
Lee and Park,[30] 2016	84	Nodules, polyps, Reinke edema	2 y	44% complete remission; 26% partial remission; 23% recurrence (average time was 8.2 mo); Jitter, Shimmer, VHI, grade of mucosal wave remained stable through 24 mo	1.1% hematoma rate; 1.1% prolonged white plaques
Wang et al,[52] 2017	189	Nodules, polyps, cysts	2 y	75% positive response initially; 50% continue to have positive effect at 24 mo; 12%, 17%, 24%, and 32% failure rate at 6, 12, 18, and 24 mo, respectively	Not reported

Abbreviations: GRB, global, roughness, breathiness scale; GRBAS, grade, roughness, breathiness, asthenia, strain scale; HNR, harmonic-to-noise ratio; MPT, maximal phonation time; VAS, visual analog scale; VHI, voice handicap index.

TECHNICAL DETAILS
Steroid Formulations

A variety of corticosteroids have been used for VFSI. Studies suggest that triamcinolone has a longer duration, with dexamethasone having greater anti-inflammatory effects.[26,27,29] Triamcinolone leaves a white plaque appearance to the vocal fold that typically subsides after a few months.[30,31] **Table 4** lists commonly used steroids and doses.

Approaches

VFSI uses the same approaches as vocal fold augmentation. It is critical to visualize the needle entering the base of the lesion. The amount of steroid injected varies (see **Table 3**). Injection deep into the superficial lamina propria should be avoided to prevent thyroarytenoid muscle atrophy (**Fig. 3**). Post-operative care is the same as in vocal fold augmentation, although some surgeons advocate for a short period of voice rest of 3 days.

Complications

Complications from VFSI tends are minor and rare. The most common reported complications include vocal fold hematoma (<2%), white subepithelial plaques, and vocal fold atrophy.[30,31]

SPASMODIC DYSPHONIA
Introduction

Spasmodic dysphonia (SD) is a focal dystonia that results from involuntary vocal fold spasms divided into adductor SD (ADSD), abductor SD (ABSD), and mixed SD.[32] Adductor SD accounts for 80% of SD, with the remaining 20% split between ABSD and mixed.[33] Diagnosis is made on auditory-perceptual evaluation and spasmodic activity on flexible laryngoscopy.[32] Adductor SD patients typically exhibit abrupt initiation and termination of voicing, resulting in short breaks in phonation. Symptoms are typically worsened when under stress and improve in the morning or after an alcoholic drink. Classically, patients may laugh and sing without phonation breaks. Patients with ABSD exhibit a breathy and effortful voice with abrupt termination by aphonic, whispered segments.[34] Laryngeal botulinum toxin (BTX) injections are the current standard of care for SD, lasting approximately 3 months. Antibody formation against BTX in laryngeal applications is extraordinarily rare owing the low number of units

Table 4		
Quantity/formulation of steroids for VFSI		
Study	**Steroid**	**Quantity**
Hsu et al,[51] 2009	Triamcinolone acetonide (40 mg/mL)	0.1 mL per lesion
Mortensen and Woo,[25] 2006	Methylprednisolone acetate suspension (40 mg/mL), USP	Not reported
Woo et al,[31] 2011	Triamcinolone acetonide (40 mg/mL)	0.15–0.2 mL per lesion
Wang et al,[29] 2013	0.1 mL of dexamethasone sodium phosphate (4 mg/mL)	0.1 mL per lesion
Wang et al,[26] 2015	1:1 mixture of triamcinolone acetonide (10 mg/mL) and dexamethasone sodium phosphate (5 mg/mL)	0.1–1.0 mL per lesion
Lee and Park,[30] 2016	Triamcinolone acetonide (40 mg/mL)	Not reported

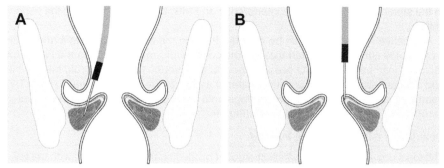

Fig. 3. (*A*) Needle location within the vocal fold for injection augmentation into the muscle. (*B*) Needle location with the tip in the superficial lamina propria for vocal fold steroid injections. Both illustrations depict a sheathed needle through a channeled flexible laryngoscope.

required for treatment.[34] Contraindications to laryngeal BTX use include pregnancy, lactation, pre-existing neuromuscular disorders (eg, myasthenia gravis, Eaton-Lambert disease), and patients taking aminoglycosides.[34]

Technique

There are 2 primary approaches to laryngeal botox injection: electromyography (EMG)-guided and non-EMG guided. Location and amount of injection depends on the technique in addition to the type of SD.

Adductor Spasmodic Dysphonia

Patients lie back in the examination chair with their neck extended for EMG-guided BTX injections. Local anesthetics are sometimes avoided because of possible interference with EMG-guided injection. Doses of 1% lidocaine with 1:100,000 epinephrine can be injected into the skin over the cricothyroid membrane. A monopolar hollow polytetrafluoroethylene (Teflon)-coated EMG needle is inserted through the cricothyroid membrane in the midline and then directed approximately 30° superiorly and laterally until the desired muscle activity is identified on EMG. The patient can be instructed to say /i/ to augment this response and confirm needle location followed by injection of BTX.

A per-oral or thyrohyoid approach, similar to augmentation targeting the thyroarytenoid muscle injection, is an alternative option if an EMG machine is unavailable, although some reports suggest that this approach is less accurate.[34] Another option is injection into the submucosa of each supraglottic fold without the use of EMG guidance.[32] Similarly, transnasal endoscopic injections are performed, although they have the disadvantage of priming the long needle sheath, wasting approximately 50 units of BTX.[35] Patients with mixed SD require a combination of BTX injections.

Abductor Spasmodic Dysphonia

ABSD requires posterior cricoarytenoid muscle BTX injection and is technically more challenging. The patient is positioned the same as for ADSD injections, and the larynx is rotated away from the side of the planned injection. The EMG needle is directed toward the posterior edge of the thyroid lamina at the junction of the superior two-thirds and inferior one-third of the thyroid cartilage, with the needle penetrating the inferior constrictor muscle and abutting the cricoid cartilage.[35] The needle is then positioned to the area of maximum muscle interference on EMG, enhanced by having the patient sniff.

Alternatively, the needle can be directed through the cricothyroid membrane, with 1 mL of 4% lidocaine injected through the cricothyroid membrane into the larynx for topical anesthesia. The EMG needle is positioned through the cricothyroid membrane and directed slightly lateral until the posterior aspect to the cricoid cartilage is felt. The needle is advanced through the cartilage until EMG cricoarytenoid muscle signal is recognized, and BTX is administered (**Fig. 4**).[34]

Quantity of Botulinum Toxin Injected

The ideal dose of BTX is the smallest amount producing the most benefit with the fewest side effects, and is patient specific. A starting dose of 1.0 units unilaterally or bilaterally in patients with ADSD is reasonable or performing opposite side injection 2 weeks after the initial side to minimize breathiness.[34] For supraglottic fold injections, a starting dose of 7 units has been reported.[32] Subsequent injections are tailored to achieve maximal benefit using the lowest dose with least side effects. Experience suggests that women require more BTX than men.[36] Response for amount injected for ABSD is more variable. Blitzer and Bielamowicz in their respective studies injected 1 vocal fold initially with injection of the contralateral side 2 to 3 weeks later to prevent dyspnea or stridor.[33,35]

Outcomes

Patients with ADSD have significant subjective and objective improvement after BTX injections.[32,33,37] Outcomes for BTX in ABSD are inferior as a result of a more difficult technique and increased BTX dose resulting in dyspnea.

Complications

Breathy dysphonia is common, especially early in treatment, with a reported 50.9% breathiness rate lasting an average of 20 days.[37] A report of supraglottic fold injections without EMG guidance in 25 patients for a total of 198 injections showed that 76% did

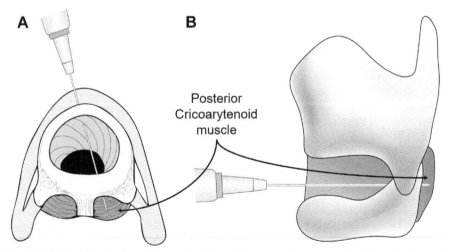

Fig. 4. (A) Axial illustration of trans-cricoid cartilage needle approach to the posterior cricoarytenoid (PCA) muscle. (B) Sagittal view of trans-cricoid cartilage botulinum toxin injection into the PCA muscle.

not have the initial dip in phonatory function.[32] Dysphagia and coughing with liquids occurs in from 2% to 15%, lasting about 2 weeks.[37] Failure to improve occurs in about 30% regardless of technique.[38] For ABSD, over-injection, particularly to bilateral posterior cricoarytenoid muscles, can result in stridor, requiring tracheotomy.[34] Minor wheezing or stridor occurs in 2.5% of patients, and dysphagia in another 6.5%, in ABSD or mixed therapy.[34]

OFFICE-BASED CHRONIC COUGH TREATMENT

Cough persisting beyond 8 weeks is termed chronic cough, with etiologies ranging from postnasal drip, asthma, gastroesophageal reflux disease, and angiotensin converting enzyme inhibitor use.[39] When cough persists with treatment of these etiologies, it is termed idiopathic cough, habit cough, psychogenic cough, neurogenic cough, or hypersensitivity cough syndrome. Neuromodulating agents, such as tricyclic antidepressants, baclofen, tramadol, and gabapentin have been used with varying results.[39,40] Botulinum toxin, superior laryngeal nerve injections, and injection laryngoplasty demonstrate some benefit.

Botulinum toxin treatment of chronic cough targets the thyroarytenoid muscles to disrupt and reduce the cough pathway, with some studies finding improvement in at least 50% of patients.[41] Recently, superior laryngeal nerve injections with triamcinolone acetonide and a local anesthetic improved symptoms in most patients.[42] In addition, patients with chronic cough and nerve paresis who underwent carboxymethycellulose injection augmentation had decreased cough severity.[43]

SUMMARY

Application and frequency of office-based laryngeal injections continue to expand with improving videolaryngoscopy equipment, increased supporting literature, and the potential for avoiding general anesthesia, shorter procedural times, and decreased costs. Surgeons may select from a variety of approaches and materials for vocal fold augmentation and VFSIs to accommodate for available equipment, patient anatomy, patient comfort, and surgeon experience. Recent evidence also suggests a role for a variety of laryngeal injections for neurogenic cough. There are also in-office SD BTX injection approaches with or without EMG guidance. Familiarity with the breadth of available in-office laryngeal injections allows otolaryngologists to optimize, tailor, and administer treatment for an expanding cohort of laryngeal conditions in the office setting.

REFERENCES

1. Verma SP, Dailey SH. Office-based injection laryngoplasty for the management of unilateral vocal fold paralysis. J Voice 2014;28(3):382–6.
2. Marcus S, Timen M, Dion GR, et al. Cost analysis of channeled, distal chip laryngoscope for in-office laryngopharyngeal biopsies. J Voice 2018. [Epub ahead of print].
3. Rosen CA, Amin MR, Sulica L, et al. Advances in office-based diagnosis and treatment in laryngology. Laryngoscope 2009;119(Suppl 2):S185–212.
4. Milstein CF, Akst LM, Hicks MD, et al. Long-term effects of micronized Alloderm injection for unilateral vocal fold paralysis. Laryngoscope 2005;115(9):1691–6.
5. King JM, Simpson CB. Modern injection augmentation for glottic insufficiency. Curr Opin Otolaryngol Head Neck Surg 2007;15(3):153–8.

6. Sulica L, Rosen CA, Postma GN, et al. Current practice in injection augmentation of the vocal folds: indications, treatment principles, techniques, and complications. Laryngoscope 2010;120(2):319–25.

7. Damrose EJ. Percutaneous injection laryngoplasty in the management of acute vocal fold paralysis. Laryngoscope 2010;120(8):1582–90.

8. Dion GR, Achlatis E, Teng S, et al. Changes in peak airflow measurement during maximal cough after vocal fold augmentation in patients with glottic insufficiency. JAMA Otolaryngol Head Neck Surg 2017;143(11):1141–5.

9. Reiter R, Brosch S. Laryngoplasty with hyaluronic acid in patients with unilateral vocal fold paralysis. J Voice 2012;26(6):785–91.

10. Mallur PS, Rosen CA. Office-based laryngeal injections. Otolaryngol Clin North Am 2013;46(1):85–100.

11. Kwon TK, Buckmire R. Injection laryngoplasty for management of unilateral vocal fold paralysis. Curr Opin Otolaryngol Head Neck Surg 2004;12(6):538–42.

12. Mohammed H, Masterson L, Gendy S, et al. Outpatient-based injection laryngoplasty for the management of unilateral vocal fold paralysis - clinical outcomes from a UK centre. Clin Otolaryngol 2016;41(4):341–6.

13. Woo SH, Son YI, Lee SH, et al. Comparative analysis on the efficiency of the injection laryngoplasty technique using calcium hydroxyapatite (CaHA): the thyrohyoid approach versus the cricothyroid approach. J Voice 2013;27(2):236–41.

14. Woo P. Office-based laryngeal procedures. Otolaryngol Clin North Am 2006; 39(1):111–33.

15. Taleb M, Ashraf Z, Valavoor S, et al. Evaluation and management of acquired methemoglobinemia associated with topical benzocaine use. Am J Cardiovasc Drugs 2013;13(5):325–30.

16. Amin MR. Thyrohyoid approach for vocal fold augmentation. Ann Otol Rhinol Laryngol 2006;115(9):699–702.

17. O'Leary MA, Grillone GA. Injection laryngoplasty. Otolaryngol Clin North Am 2006;39(1):43–54.

18. Trask DK, Shellenberger DL, Hoffman HT. Transnasal, endoscopic vocal fold augmentation. Laryngoscope 2005;115(12):2262–5.

19. Ford CN, Bless DM, Loftus JM. Role of injectable collagen in the treatment of glottic insufficiency: a study of 119 patients. Ann Otol Rhinol Laryngol 1992;101(3): 237–47.

20. Bock JM, Lee JH, Robinson RA, et al. Migration of Cymetra after vocal fold injection for laryngeal paralysis. Laryngoscope 2007;117(12):2251–4.

21. Carroll TL, Rosen CA. Long-term results of calcium hydroxylapatite for vocal fold augmentation. Laryngoscope 2011;121(2):313–9.

22. Ting JY, Patel R, Halum SL. Managing voice impairment after injection laryngoplasty. J Voice 2012;26(6):797–800.

23. DeFatta RA, Chowdhury FR, Sataloff RT. Complications of injection laryngoplasty using calcium hydroxylapatite. J Voice 2012;26(5):614–8.

24. Young WG, Hoffman MR, Koszewski IJ, et al. Voice outcomes following a single office-based steroid injection for vocal fold scar. Otolaryngol Head Neck Surg 2016;155(5):820–8.

25. Mortensen M, Woo P. Office steroid injections of the larynx. Laryngoscope 2006; 116(10):1735–9.

26. Wang CT, Lai MS, Hsiao TY. Comprehensive outcome researches of intralesional steroid injection on benign vocal fold lesions. J Voice 2015;29(5):578–87.

27. Wang CT, Liao LJ, Cheng PW, et al. Intralesional steroid injection for benign vocal fold disorders: a systematic review and meta-analysis. Laryngoscope 2013; 123(1):197–203.

28. Wang CT, Liao LJ, Lai MS, et al. Comparison of benign lesion regression following vocal fold steroid injection and vocal hygiene education. Laryngoscope 2014; 124(2):510–5.

29. Wang CT, Lai MS, Liao LJ, et al. Transnasal endoscopic steroid injection: a practical and effective alternative treatment for benign vocal fold disorders. Laryngoscope 2013;123(6):1464–8.

30. Lee SW, Park KN. Long-term efficacy of percutaneous steroid injection for treating benign vocal fold lesions: a prospective study. Laryngoscope 2016;126(10): 2315–9.

31. Woo JH, Kim DY, Kim JW, et al. Efficacy of percutaneous vocal fold injections for benign laryngeal lesions: prospective multicenter study. Acta Otolaryngol 2011; 131(12):1326–32.

32. Simpson CB, Lee CT, Hatcher JL, et al. Botulinum toxin treatment of false vocal folds in adductor spasmodic dysphonia: functional outcomes. Laryngoscope 2016;126(1):118–21.

33. Blitzer A, Brin MF, Stewart CF. Botulinum toxin management of spasmodic dysphonia (laryngeal dystonia): a 12-year experience in more than 900 patients. Laryngoscope 1998;108(10):1435–41.

34. Gibbs SR, Blitzer A. Botulinum toxin for the treatment of spasmodic dysphonia. Otolaryngol Clin North Am 2000;33(4):879–94.

35. Bielamowicz S, Squire S, Bidus K, et al. Assessment of posterior cricoarytenoid botulinum toxin injections in patients with abductor spasmodic dysphonia. Ann Otol Rhinol Laryngol 2001;110(5 Pt 1):406–12.

36. Lerner MZ, Lerner BA, Patel AA, et al. Gender differences in onabotulinum toxin A dosing for adductor spasmodic dysphonia. Laryngoscope 2017;127(5):1131–4.

37. Novakovic D, Waters HH, D'Elia JB, et al. Botulinum toxin treatment of adductor spasmodic dysphonia: longitudinal functional outcomes. Laryngoscope 2011; 121(3):606–12.

38. Galardi G, Guerriero R, Amadio S, et al. Sporadic failure of botulinum toxin treatment in usually responsive patients with adductor spasmodic dysphonia. Neurol Sci 2001;22(4):303–6.

39. Sasieta HC, Iyer VN, Orbelo DM, et al. Bilateral thyroarytenoid botulinum toxin type A injection for the treatment of refractory chronic cough. JAMA Otolaryngol Head Neck Surg 2016;142(9):881–8.

40. Dion GR, Teng SE, Achlatis E, et al. Treatment of neurogenic cough with tramadol: a pilot study. Otolaryngol Head Neck Surg 2017;157(1):77–9.

41. Chu MW, Lieser JD, Sinacori JT. Use of botulinum toxin type A for chronic cough: a neuropathic model. Arch Otolaryngol Head Neck Surg 2010;136(5):447–52.

42. Simpson CB, Tibbetts KM, Loochtan MJ, et al. Treatment of chronic neurogenic cough with in-office superior laryngeal nerve block. Laryngoscope 2018;128(8): 1898–903.

43. Crawley BK, Murry T, Sulica L. Injection augmentation for chronic cough. J Voice 2015;29(6):763–7.

44. Courey MS. Injection laryngoplasty. Otolaryngol Clin North Am 2004;37(1): 121–38.

45. Anderson TD, Sataloff RT. Complications of collagen injection of the vocal fold: report of several unusual cases and review of the literature. J Voice 2004;18(3): 392–7.

46. Zapanta PE, Bielamowicz SA. Laryngeal abscess after injection laryngoplasty with micronized AlloDerm. Laryngoscope 2004;114(9):1522–4.

47. Tanna N, Zalkind D, Glade RS, et al. Foreign body reaction to calcium hydroxyl-apatite vocal fold augmentation. Arch Otolaryngol Head Neck Surg 2006; 132(12):1379–82.

48. Dominguez LM, Tibbetts KM, Simpson CB. Inflammatory reaction to hyaluronic acid: a newly described complication in vocal fold augmentation. Laryngoscope 2017;127(2):445–9.

49. Tateya I, Omori K, Kojima H, et al. Steroid injection for Reinke's edema using fiber-optic laryngeal surgery. Acta Otolaryngol 2003;123(3):417–20.

50. Tateya I, Omori K, Kojima H, et al. Steroid injection to vocal nodules using fiber-optic laryngeal surgery under topical anesthesia. Eur Arch Otorhinolaryngol 2004;261(9):489–92.

51. Hsu YB, Lan MC, Chang SY. Percutaneous corticosteroid injection for vocal fold polyp. Arch Otolaryngol Head Neck Surg 2009;135(8):776–80.

52. Wang CT, Lai MS, Cheng PW. Long-term surveillance following intralesional steroid injection for benign vocal fold lesions. JAMA Otolaryngol Head Neck Surg 2017;143(6):589–94.

Office-Based 532-Nanometer Pulsed Potassium-Titanyl-Phosphate Laser Procedures in Laryngology

Kathleen M. Tibbetts, MD[a],*, Charles Blakely Simpson, MD[b]

KEYWORDS

- Potassium-titanyl-phosphate laser • Office-based procedures
- Office-based laser surgery • Laryngology • Benign laryngeal lesions
- Recurrent respiratory papillomatosis

KEY POINTS

- Advances in technology have led to the expansion of in-office procedures in laryngology. The potassium-titanyl-phosphate (KTP) laser, because of its absorption by oxyhemoglobin and fiber-based delivery system, is ideal for in-office laryngeal laser surgery.
- In-office KTP laser procedures under topical anesthesia have been shown to be safe and effective when compared with similar procedures in the operating room setting under general anesthesia.
- The KTP laser may be used for treatment of recurrent respiratory papillomatosis, leukoplakia, and dysplasia, and other benign laryngeal lesions, such as polyps and granulomas. New indications for in-office KTP laser procedures continue to appear in the literature.

 Video content accompanies this article at http://www.oto.theclinics.com.

INTRODUCTION

Advances in technology, availability of equipment, changes in patient demographics, and efforts to decrease health care costs have led to the expansion of in-office procedures in recent years. This change is particularly true within laryngology, and many procedures for management of laryngeal pathology traditionally performed in the operating room are now routinely performed in the office setting. The publication

Disclosure Statement: Dr. Simpson is a consultant for Olympus. Dr. Tibbetts has no disclosures.
[a] Department of Otolaryngology-Head and Neck Surgery, University of Texas Southwestern Medical Center, 2001 Inwood Road, 7th Floor, Dallas, TX 75390, USA; [b] Department of Otolaryngology-Head and Neck Surgery, University of Texas Voice Center, University of Texas Health Science Center-San Antonio, 8431 Fredricksburg Road, San Antonio, TX 78229, USA
* Corresponding author.
E-mail address: Kathleen.tibbetts@utsouthwestern.edu

Otolaryngol Clin N Am 52 (2019) 537–557
https://doi.org/10.1016/j.otc.2019.02.011
0030-6665/19/© 2019 Elsevier Inc. All rights reserved.

Abbreviations	
AT	Antithrombotic
CO_2	Carbon dioxide
GRBAS	Grade of hoarseness, roughness, breathiness, asthenia, and strain
HPV	Human papillomavirus
KTP	Potassium-titanyl-phosphate
NPO	Nil per os
NSAID	Nonsteroidal anti-inflammatory drug
PDL	Pulsed dye laser
Pps	Pulses per second
RRP	Recurrent respiratory papillomatosis
VHI-10	Voice Handicap Index-10

of methods for topical anesthetization of the upper aerodigestive tract and techniques for in-office laryngeal procedures helped begin the trend toward the management of laryngeal pathology in the office setting.[1,2] The improved visualization provided by distal chip flexible endoscopes has allowed for better visual delineation of lesions and increased precision of treatment. The development of new injection materials and fiber-based lasers allowed for rapid expansion these procedures over the last several years.[3] Performing laryngeal surgery in the office setting has obvious advantages, including avoidance of general anesthesia and the associated risks. In-office procedures also offer shorter recovery times and significantly lower costs than similar procedures performed in the operating room.

For decades, lasers have advanced otolaryngologic surgery, with the carbon dioxide (CO_2), argon, and dye lasers being some of the earliest used.[4] The addition of the neodymium:yttrium-aluminum-garnet, potassium-titanyl-phosphate (KTP), and holmium lasers further broadened the indications for laser surgery. The choice of laser depends on wavelength, the characteristics of the target tissue, and the energy density of the laser. The CO_2 laser was the first to be used in the larynx and upper airway for a variety of conditions including benign and malignant lesions.[5] The CO_2 laser energy is absorbed by water, which has a high concentration in laryngeal tissues. It can be coupled to a microscope allowing magnification and precise control of the aiming beam via a micromanipulator.[4] Because the CO_2 laser was initially limited to mirror-reflected line of sight delivery, its application to laryngeal surgery was initially only via direct laryngoscopy in the operating room under general anesthesia.

Office-based laser surgery in otolaryngology was first described in 2001, and used the 585-nm pulsed dye laser (PDL) under topical anesthesia. Features of the PDL laser that made it advantageous for in-office laryngeal procedures included its fiber delivery system and its energy's selective absorption by oxyhemoglobin, which made it suitable for treatment of vascular lesions, such as recurrent respiratory papillomatosis (RRP).[6] Several disadvantages of the PDL became apparent, however, particularly procedural bleeding caused by the laser's short pulse width of approximately 0.5 ms, and the large size of the fiber (0.6 mm). The fiber size resulted in damage to the working channels of laryngoscopes and difficulty with suctioning during the procedure.[7]

The shortcomings of the PDL led to the use of the pulsed KTP laser for in-office laryngeal surgery, first described by Zeitels and colleagues[7] in 2006. The investigators noted that the wavelength of the KTP laser (532 nm) is more absorbable by oxyhemoglobin, and the extended pulse width (15 ms) allows for distribution of energy over a longer time period. This results in more effective intravascular coagulation via slower intraluminal heating, and avoids photothermal injury to the superficial lamina propria.[8]

The smaller fiber size of 0.2 or 0.4 mm is another advantage of the KTP laser,[4] which allows more efficient suctioning and improved visualization.

In the office setting, the KTP laser was first applied to vascular glottic epithelial lesions (dysplasia and RRP), targeting their microcirculation.[7] Later investigations, including a multi-institutional study published in 2012, have shown the KTP laser to be effective in the treatment of nonvascular benign laryngeal lesions, such as Reinke edema and leukoplakia. The authors hypothesized that nonspecific thermal injury to adjacent target chromophores, such as blood vessels, results in wound repair that leads to lesion regression.[9] The indications for office-based KTP laser laryngeal surgery have continued to expand, and it has grown in popularity with surgeons and patients.

EQUIPMENT AND SUPPLIES

The most crucial piece of equipment for in-office laser procedures is the laser itself. The Aura XP pulsed-KTP laser system (Aura KTP, Boston Scientific, Marlborough, MA) is the most widely used within laryngology practices (**Fig. 1**A). The Aura KTP laser has a wavelength of 532 nm, power of 0.5 to 15 W, and peak power of 160 W. The system may be purchased new or used, or rented through a mobile surgical technology service. Its compact size (dimensions of 42 cm × 31 cm × 58 cm, weight 27 kg) allows for accommodation in most examination or procedure rooms. Single-use laser fibers are required (EndoStat Fiber, Boston Scientific), and range in diameter from 0.2 mm to 0.6 mm, with lengths of 12 or 18 feet. Protective eyewear specific to the KTP laser wavelength is required for all personnel and the patient (KTP/532 Plastic Protective Glasses, Boston Scientific) (**Fig. 1**B).

A channeled laryngoscope is another critical piece of equipment for in-office laser procedures. The authors use the ENF-VT2 channeled rhinolaryngoscope (Olympus, Center Valley, PA). The working side channel is necessary for passage of the laser fiber, and may be used to administer topical anesthesia. A disposable catheter with a Luer-lock attachment is passed via the side channel, and the anesthetic administered via a syringe (flexible suction catheter with Luer-lock, Karl Storz Endoscopy-America, Inc, El Segundo, CA) (**Fig. 1**C). Similar nondisposable catheters (Washing Pipe PW-6P-1, Olympus) are available and may be sterilized and reprocessed in between procedures. A metal sheath (MAJ-655, Olympus) is passed through the working channel of the laryngoscope before insertion of the laser fiber; this protects the laryngoscope against damage from the fiber. The other necessary supplies for the procedure are available in most otolaryngology clinics: a decongestant and local anesthetic for preparation of the nasal cavity (oxymetazoline plus 1% lidocaine or 2% tetracaine), and 4% lidocaine for topical anesthetization of the larynx.

At some centers, the KTP laser and other necessary equipment may be owned and managed by a surgery center or endoscopy facility. Differences in billing and reimbursement for facility versus nonfacility awake KTP laser procedures are discussed later.

PATIENT SELECTION

In planning for laryngeal surgery on awake patients, tolerance of the procedure is an obvious consideration. In general, in-office laryngeal procedures are well tolerated by most patients. Rees and colleagues[10] surveyed patients who had undergone unsedated in-office PDL laryngeal procedures, and found an average comfort score of 7.4 (scale, 1–10; 10 = minimal discomfort). Eighty-seven percent of patients stated that they would prefer in-office procedures to surgery under general anesthesia.

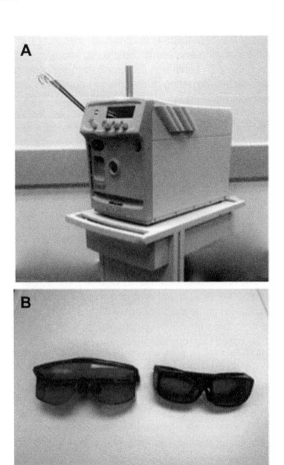

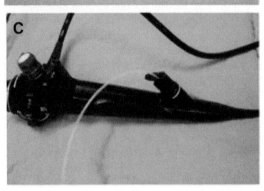

Fig. 1. Equipment necessary for in-office KTP laser procedures. (*A*) Aura XP pulsed-KTP laser system (Aura KTP, Boston Scientific, Marlborough, MA). (*B*) Protective eyewear specific to the KTP laser wavelength (KTP/532 Plastic Protective Glasses, Boston Scientific). (*C*) Channeled laryngoscope with Luer-lock catheter passed through the working channel for administration of topical anesthesia (ENF-VT2 channeled rhinolaryngoscope with side channel and Washing Pipe PW-6P-1, Olympus, Center Valley, PA).

In-office laryngeal procedures using the CO_2 laser were similarly well tolerated, with a mean pain score during the procedure of 2/10 (10 = intolerable pain).[11] Patients preferred several aspects of in-office procedures in comparison with operating room procedures: decreased time and cost of the procedure, improved convenience and comfort, and avoidance of general anesthesia.[10] In a multi-institutional study, Young and colleagues[12] explored patient tolerance of a variety of awake in-office laryngeal procedures, and factors that influenced patient tolerance. Patients reported an average of 37/100 on a discomfort scale (0 = no discomfort, 100 = maximal discomfort). Procedures were completed successfully in 92% of patients, and 93% of patients would be willing to undergo another procedure. High preprocedure anxiety did not impact patient comfort or procedure completion rate. Uncontrolled gag reflex and copious secretions were factors that resulted in difficulty with the procedure.

Based on the existing studies and the authors' experience, most patients are able to tolerate in-office laser laryngeal procedures. Patients with a strong gag reflex may need extra topical anesthesia or nebulized lidocaine. Patients with poor tolerance of the initial laryngeal examination with a rhinolaryngoscope or rigid endoscope may be deemed poor candidates for in-office procedures, or may not wish to pursue them because of anticipated discomfort. Nasal patency is another consideration in planning in-office KTP laryngeal procedures. The outer diameter of the laryngoscope with working side channel is 4.9 mm. Therefore, the patient must have nasal passage with adequate patency to accommodate that diameter. Placement of neuropatties soaked in oxymetazoline and lidocaine/tetracaine in the nasal cavity for several minutes before the procedure is sometimes helpful with smaller nasal vaults.

In patients with significant anxiety, a low-dose anxiolytic medication may be prescribed and self-administered approximately 30 to 60 minutes before the procedure. If the procedure is performed in a surgery center, intravenous anxiolytics and/or mild sedation administered by an anesthesiologist may be an option. A recent study by Anderson and colleagues[13] found that 70% of patients who could not tolerate an initial in-office KTP laser procedure were able to complete a subsequent procedure with premedication with lorazepam 30 to 60 minutes before the procedure.

From a general health and comorbidity standpoint, there are few contraindications to awake in-office laryngeal surgery, although patients with comorbidities may require special considerations. Multiple studies have examined the physiologic changes that take place in patients undergoing awake in-office procedures. Yung and Courey[14] studied hemodynamic changes in 31 patients undergoing office-based flexible endoscopic surgery, including vocal fold injection, transnasal esophagoscopy, KTP and CO_2 laser procedures, and flexible laryngoscopy with biopsy. Twenty-nine percent of patients experienced tachycardia and 23% of patients developed severe hypertension during the procedure. They found a mean increase in heart rate of 14.6 beats per minute, a mean increase in diastolic blood pressure of 18.5 mm Hg, a mean increase in systolic blood pressure of 33.1 mm Hg, and a mean change in oxygen saturation of 0.8%. Older patients and patients with existing cardiovascular comorbidities did not have greater changes in blood pressure compared with younger patients and those without comorbidities, but their baseline blood pressures were higher, placing them at greater risk for severely elevated blood pressure during the procedure. The authors suggested that clinicians consider monitoring vital signs during in-office procedures to prevent potential cardiovascular complications.[14]

Similarly, Morrison and colleagues[15] studied hemodynamic changes in 100 patients undergoing awake office-based flexible endoscopic procedures. They found that severe hypertension occurred in 21% of patients, and tachycardia in 40%. In patients older than 50 years of age and those undergoing esophageal or laser procedures, there were statistically significant elevations in heart rate. Patients undergoing esophageal or laser procedures also had a statistically significant elevation in diastolic blood pressure. The authors suggested monitoring vital signs in patients older than 50 years of age, and those who may be at risk for cardiovascular complications undergoing esophageal or laser procedures.

Although studies have shown that hemodynamic changes do occur in patients undergoing in-office procedures, there is evidence that these may be less than those that occur under general anesthesia. Tierney and colleagues[16] compared heart rate and blood pressure measurements of patients undergoing laryngeal surgery in the operating room and in the clinic setting. The authors found that severe hemodynamic events, specifically tachycardia or hypertension (blood pressure >180 mm Hg systolic or >110 mm Hg diastolic) occurred significantly more frequently in the operating room than in the office (41% vs 20%, respectively). The authors concluded that for procedures that may be performed in either setting, there may be a safety benefit to performing them in the office.

Recently, a preprocedure screening protocol was developed and applied to patients undergoing awake in-office laryngeal procedures. Madden and colleagues[17] screened 440 patients by measuring heart rate and blood pressure. If vital signs were within the set parameters (heart rate <100 beats per minute, systolic blood pressure <160 mm Hg, diastolic blood pressure <100 mg Hg), the procedure was performed in the office setting. Patients with elevations in heart rate and blood pressure on the screening examination were referred to their primary care physician for medical management of tachycardia and/or hypertension before the procedure. If vital signs were within parameters the day of procedure after medical management, it was performed in the office, and if not, it was rescheduled and performed in a monitored setting. There were no hemodynamic complications that occurred during the study. Overall, previous studies suggest that in-office laryngeal procedures can be performed safely for most patients, but those with cardiovascular comorbidities should be closely screened and potentially monitored to prevent complications.

TREATMENT GOALS

The primary goal of in-office KTP laser procedures is to induce resolution of the target lesions while avoiding the need for management in the operating room. In addition to voice preservation, specific treatment goals are dependent on the lesion in question. For example, in the case of laryngeal papilloma, the goal is to control disease with the expectation that lesions will recur, whereas with dysplasia the goal is disease regression.[7] In the office setting, treatment time is limited by the duration of topical anesthesia. To avoid toxicity, the maximum dose of lidocaine must not be exceeded (3–5 mg/kg),[18] and lidocaine in any form has a half-life of 90 minutes.[19] Therefore, re-administering lidocaine after the initial dosage has worn off is unsafe because of risk of toxicity, so procedure time is limited by length of anesthesia provided by the initially administered lidocaine. Because of this time constraint, patients should be counseled that more than one treatment may be required for adequate treatment if the desired effect is not achieved during the first procedure. If the disease burden is anticipated to be too great to be managed by in-office procedures, or poor patient tolerance of the procedure limits operative time, scheduling the subsequent procedure in the operating room may be prudent.

PRETREATMENT PLANNING

Preprocedure instructions and counseling are paramount to ensuring safe and effective in-office laryngeal procedures. A discussion of the steps and details of the procedure may be helpful in reducing anxiety in some patients. Because no anesthesia is administered, patients are not required to be nil per os (NPO), but the authors typically recommend avoiding a large meal before the procedure to avoid gastrointestinal upset and/or vomiting if gagging occurs during the procedure. It is helpful to inform patients of any post-procedure precautions and restrictions so that they may plan accordingly. For example, patients should be informed that they will need to remain NPO for 1 to 2 hours after the procedure, and informed of any voice conservation or rest that are recommended.

Patients treated with antithrombotic (AT) medical therapy may be asked to hold these medications before the procedure, but this may be based on the surgeon's preference. AT medications have not been shown to increase the rate of complications or impact treatment outcomes of in-office laryngeal procedures. Fritz and colleagues[20] retrospectively reviewed 127 in-office laryngeal procedures, in which 27 patients were on AT medications that were not held before the procedure. The cohort included patients undergoing KTP laser procedures, and vocal fold injection augmentation, laryngeal biopsy, and injection of steroid or cidofovir. Minimal or no bleeding was reported for all procedures, and there were no postoperative complications in patients on AT medications. AT medications also did not have an adverse effect on outcomes, measured in change in Voice Handicap Index-10 scores. It is likely safe to proceed with in-office laryngeal procedures in patients on AT therapy, but holding these medications would certainly be acceptable practice.

Patients with significant anxiety surrounding the procedure may be prescribed a low-dose anxiolytic to be taken 30 to 60 minutes before the appointment. Those patients need to arrange for transportation to and from the procedure to avoid driving while under the influence of these medications.

PATIENT POSITIONING AND ANESTHESIA

Patients are positioned seated in the upright position for in-office KTP laser laryngeal procedures. In the office setting, they may be seated in a standard examination chair (**Fig. 2**). If the procedure is performed in a surgery center or endoscopy suite, they may be seated on a stretcher, operating table, or chair.

Anesthesia is topical, beginning with decongestion and anesthesia of the nasal cavity. Both nasal passages are decongested and anesthetized, unless there is an anatomic reason that one nasal passage is inaccessible, such as a severely deviated

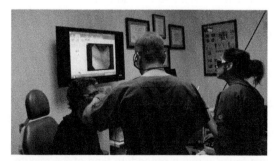

Fig. 2. Patient positioning and equipment set up for in-office KTP laser procedures. The patient is seated in the upright position in the examination chair, and the flexible channeled laryngoscope with laser fiber is passed through the most patent nasal passage. An assistant activates the laser once the fiber is positioned above the target pathology, and the surgeon fires the laser using a foot pedal.

septum. Topical oxymetazoline is used for decongestion, followed by a topical local anesthetic, such as 2% tetracaine. Two percent lidocaine may also be used, but the amount must be considered when calculating the maximum dose of lidocaine for the patient.

The laryngopharyngeal complex may then be anesthetized either via a transnasal or transoral approach. With the transnasal approach, 4% lidocaine is administered via the working channel of the laryngoscope (Video 1). A catheter with Luer lock may be passed via the working channel, and the syringe of lidocaine attached to this. A total of 6 mL is typically adequate for anesthesia for therapeutic procedures, such as KTP laser treatment, and only 3 mL is necessary for diagnostic studies, such as tracheobronchscopy.[18] The patient is asked to phonate (hold a long E) during administration of lidocaine to the vocal folds to produce a "laryngeal gargle."[21] If evaluation of treatment of lesions within the tracheobronchial tree is planned, the patient is asked to breathe while lidocaine is dripped through the vocal folds.

Although administration of 4% lidocaine via the working channel of the laryngoscope is the most straightforward method for inducing topical anesthesia during in-office KTP laser procedures, a transoral approach as initially described by Hogikyan[21] is possible. The oropharynx is anesthetized with cetacaine spray (13% benzocaine/2% butamben/2% tetracaine), and the nasal cavity is anesthetized as previously described. A flexible laryngoscope is used for visualization as 4% lidocaine is dripped onto the tongue base, supraglottis, and larynx via an Abraham cannula or a laryngotracheal atomizer spray device (MAD 600, Wolfe Tory Medical, Salt Lake City, UT). Drawbacks to this approach are that it requires an assistant to operate the endoscope, and may not be tolerated by patients with a strong gag reflex. A third option for topically anesthetizing the laryngopharyngeal complex is inhaled lidocaine via nebulization. When adequate anesthesia is achieved, most patients experience the sensation that the throat is "swollen," and swallowing may feel effortful.[22]

When administering local anesthetics, the clinician must be mindful of the maximum dosages for each particular patient to avoid toxicity. The maximum dose of lidocaine is 3 to 5 mg/kg. Four percent lidocaine is 40 mg/mL of lidocaine, and therefore 5 mL of 4% lidocaine contains 200 mg of lidocaine. To avoid toxicity, 70-kg patient may receive only up to 300 mg of lidocaine.[18] Tetracaine toxicity has been described, but at doses greater than 100 mg.[23] For in-office procedures, typically only 0.1 to 0.2 mL of 2% tetracaine is administered via an atomizer.

TECHNICAL DETAILS

After the patient is positioned and topical anesthesia is administered as described previously, the procedure may commence immediately. The authors recommend allowing as little time as possible between the completion of topical anesthesia and beginning the procedure to maximize the procedure time. Generally, no more than 60 to 90 seconds are needed after anesthetic administration is completed. In the authors' experience, patients are adequately anesthetized to tolerate KTP laser procedures for a maximum of approximately 12 minutes. A study of 145 in-office KTP laser laryngeal procedures found a mean procedure time of 6.4 minutes, with a range of 1 to 18 minutes.[13]

The channeled laryngoscope is connected to suction, and a protective metal sheath is passed via the working channel. The KTP laser fiber is passed through the protective sheath. Before passing the sheath and KTP laser fiber through the tip of the endoscope, the laryngoscope is passed via the patient's most patent nasal passage, advanced to the hypopharynx, and positioned superior to the target lesions. The sheath is then passed beyond the tip of the endoscope, and the laser fiber is then advanced distal to the tip of the sheath. At this point, the surgeon verbally indicates that the laser should be activated, and treatment may begin. The laser is operated via a foot pedal controlled by the surgeon. The KTP laser has three settings that may be adjusted: the power (measured in watts), pulse width (measured in milliseconds), and pulses per second. There is variation in recommended laser settings in the literature (**Table 1**)[7,9,24,25] and settings may vary based on the targeted pathology and surgeon preference.

In general, the tip of the laser fiber is positioned 2 to 4 mm above the target lesion and fired until the lesion blanches,[26] and in some cases the fiber may be placed in contact with the lesion. The exact technique and details of each procedure vary. Mallur and colleagues[24] proposed a five-point classification system for KTP laser effects on vocal fold lesions. The categories account for tissue effects and technique with regard to contact and noncontact treatment: type V (noncontact, angiolysis), type 1 (noncontact, epithelium intact), type 2 (noncontact, epithelium disruption), type 3 (select contact or noncontact, epithelial ablation without tissue removal), and type 4 (contact, epithelial ablation with tissue removal). If tissue removal is desired, lesions or portions of lesions are removed with contact by the laser fiber, or with suction via the endoscope. Video 2 shows an example of an in-office KTP laser procedure performed for management of RRP.

Once treatment has been completed or the effects of the topical anesthetic subside, the procedure is concluded. The laser fiber and sheath should be drawn back into the working channel before removal of the endoscope. The patient is then given postprocedure instructions and discharged. Patients are advised to remain NPO for 60 to 90 minutes to prevent aspiration caused by anesthesia of the laryngopharyngeal complex. They may be asked to rest or conserve their voice at the surgeon's discretion. If no anxiolytic was administered, patients may drive themselves home from the procedure, and no other activity restrictions are advised. Pain medication is rarely necessary, and typically acetaminophen is adequate if the patient experiences any soreness or discomfort.

Table 1
Suggested KTP laser settings for treatment of laryngeal lesions as reported in the literature

Authors	Laryngeal Lesions	Laser Settings
Zeitels et al,[7] 2006	Papillomatosis, keratosis with dysplasia	15 ms pulse width, 5.25 J per pulse
Sheu et al,[9] 2012	Benign laryngeal lesions (vocal fold polyps, granulomas, Reinke edema, vocal fold cyst, vocal fold scar, amyloidosis)	6–8 W, 15–25 ms pulse width
Mallur et al,[24] 2014	Vascular lesions (ectasias, varices, lesion-associated blood vessels)	20 W, 15 ms pulse width, 2 pps
	Nonvascular lesions (leukoplakia, papilloma, granulomas)	35 W, 15 ms pulse width, 2 pps
Sridharan et al,[25] 2014	Vocal fold polyps	15–20 W, 20–30 ms pulse width

Abbreviation: pps, pulses per second.

POSSIBLE COMPLICATIONS

Studies of a variety of in-office procedures have demonstrated extremely low rates of complications. A clear advantage of in-office laryngeal procedures is that they avoid the risks of general anesthesia, and common risks and complications of suspension laryngoscopy, such as injury to teeth, throat pain, tongue discomfort/paresthesia, and dysgeusia. In a review of 50 office-based injection laryngoplasties, Bové and colleagues[27] found no significant complications. Postma and colleagues[28] found only two minor complications (both self-limited vasovagal reactions) in more than 700 consecutive in-office transnasal esophagoscopies. In a review of 443 office-based laser procedures, Koufman and colleagues[29] found a minor complication rate of 0.9% and no major complications. Del Signore and colleagues[30] reviewed 382 in-office laser procedures, 56% of which used the KTP laser. They found a 4% complication rate, which included vocal fold stiffness, atrophy, and prolonged hyperemia. A recent study of 145 in-office KTP laser laryngeal procedures found a minor complication rate of 4.8% (vasovagal episodes and patient intolerance) and no major complications.[13]

Although reported complication rates are low, it is important to be aware of potential complications to prevent them. Recognizing early signs of vasovagal reactions allows the clinician to terminate the procedure and provide appropriate treatment to the patient to prevent syncope. Symptoms including nausea, sweating, lightheadedness, and paresthesias indicate impending syncope.[10,29] The procedure should be discontinued, and the patient placed in a reclined or supine position, or with the head between the legs. If syncope does occur, the patient should be maintained in the supine position until he or she regains consciousness. Vital signs should be monitored.[18]

Local anesthetic toxicity is a potentially serious complication. Lidocaine toxicity effects the central nervous system and cardiovascular system. Early symptoms of toxicity include lightheadedness and dizziness. Visual and auditory disturbances, such as tinnitus, may follow. Other excitatory symptoms may occur, including tremors, shivering, and muscle twitching. If an overdose is not recognized and treated, this progresses to generalized seizures, followed by coma and respiratory depression. Lidocaine also reduces cardiac muscle contractility and conduction because of a dose-dependent inotropic effect on cardiac muscle.[31] If lidocaine toxicity is suspected, any administration of local anesthetic should be terminated, as should the procedure. The patient should be placed on supplemental oxygen and hemodynamic monitoring should be initiated. The patient should then be transferred to a facility with anesthesia and intensive care support.[32]

Allergic reaction to lidocaine is a potential complication, although this has not been reported with topical lidocaine administration during endoscopic procedures.[18] Methemoglobinemia is another potential complication of topical anesthetic use. Methemoglobinemia occurs when hemoglobin in the ferrous state (Fe^{2+}) is oxidized to the ferric state (Fe^{3+}), in which it is unable to bind oxygen. Methemoglobinemia has been reported with lidocaine when used with benzocaine for bronchoscopy. Symptoms of methemoglobinemia include anxiety, headaches, fatigue, and coma; death may occur if untreated. It is characterized by desaturations and chocolate cyanosis, a violet or brown discoloration of the lips, ears, and mucus membranes that occurs because methemoglobin is darker in color than hemoglobin. Treatment is discontinuation of the causative medication and oxygen administration. Severe cases may be treated with methylene blue at a dose of 1 to 2 mg/kg administered intravenously.[33]

Laser injury to the patient, surgeon, or other staff is another potential complication of in-office KTP laser procedures. Injury to eyes, skin, and inadvertent injury to adjacent structures during the procedure are possible. Prevention of these complications is discussed in more detail in the following section covering safety considerations.

A theoretic complication of in-office KTP laser laryngeal procedures is laser fire. This complication has not been reported in the literature for in-office procedures, but is a well-documented complication of otolaryngologic surgery in the operating room.[34] In order for a fire to occur, three components are required: fuel, an oxidizer, and an ignition source/heat.[35] In the case of laser procedures, the laser is the source of heat; fuel may be any flammable material (eg, endotracheal tube, drapes); and oxygen may be administered via the anesthesia circuit, nasal cannula, or other sources.[34] In the case of in-office laser procedures, typically fuel and a concentrated oxygen source are not present. KTP lasers have not been implicated in operating room fires, with a recent review of 86 surgical fires in otolaryngology identifying no cases attributed to KTP laser.[34] Despite these reassuring data, surgeons should still take appropriate precautions when performing laser surgery in the operating room and office settings.

Failure to complete the planned treatment, either caused by patient intolerance or procedural difficulty (eg, size and/or location of lesion) requiring performance of the procedure in the operating room, is another potential complication. Even with successful procedures, multiple treatments may be necessary, and patients should be counseled as such. A study of 382 in-office laser procedures found that 27% of patients required multiple treatments. Patients with papilloma and leukoplakia were the most likely to require more than one procedure.[30]

SAFETY CONSIDERATIONS

Before initiating in-office laser procedures, all personnel who will work with lasers should complete laser safety training as mandated by their institution. Laser safety training and protocols may vary between institutions, and basic considerations are discussed here. The doors and windows of the room where the laser is being used should be closed and/or covered with a barrier, such as a screen or curtain to prevent those outside the room from being inadvertently exposed to the laser beam. Warning signs should be displayed conspicuously at any entrance to the room stating that the laser is in use. Typically, laser goggles specific to the wavelength of the laser used are placed outside the doors, so that any personnel who may need to enter the room during the procedure have access to appropriate eyewear.[36]

Eye protection is essential for patients and staff, and all individuals present for the procedure should wear protective goggles or glasses that provide protection against the wavelength of the KTP laser (532 nm). To prevent inadvertent injury to the patient or personnel, the laser should be active only when it has been passed through the endoscope, positioned within the laryngopharynx, and the surgeon is immediately ready to use it for treatment. The tip of the laser fiber should be visible through the end of the endoscope and protective sheath before being activated. A staff member activates the laser when advised by the surgeon, and the surgeon has control of the foot pedal, ensuring that the laser is only fired when he or she intends. The laser should never be active when the fiber is not passed through the endoscope, or when the endoscope has not yet been passed into the patient's laryngopharynx. Following these precautions prevents the laser from inadvertently being fired and potentially injuring the patient and/or staff.

OUTCOMES

The KTP laser has been used to treat a variety of pathologies in the office setting. The existing studies regarding indications and outcomes of in-office KTP laser treatment of laryngeal lesions are summarized next and in **Table 2**.

Table 2
Summary of the existing studies regarding outcomes of in-office KTP laser procedures for the management of laryngeal lesions

Lesion/Pathology	Authors/Year	Outcomes	Other Details
RRP	Zeitels et al,[7] 2006	20 patients underwent 36 successful in-office KTP laser procedures for RRP	Deemed successful based on patient tolerance Patients followed up as needed so disease regression was not assessed
	Zeitels et al,[37] 2011	Combined therapy with in-office intralesional bevacizumab (Avastin) and KTP laser treatment improved disease regression when compared with KTP laser treatment alone in 16/17 cases	
Leukoplakia/dysplasia	Zeitels et al,[7] 2006	28 patients underwent 34 successful in-office KTP laser procedures for dysplasia 75%–100% disease regression in 18 cases (62%) 50%–75% regression in 7 cases (24%) 25%–50% regression in 4 cases (14%)	
	Sheu et al,[9] 2012	Reduction in leukoplakia size after KTP laser treatment Mean lesion size (pixels) decreased from 24.49 to 8.66 at initial follow-up, and 3.67 at second follow-up	
	Koss et al,[43] 2017	46 patients underwent serial in-office KTP or PDL treatment of leukoplakia 19 patients (41.3%) had no remaining disease and 2 patients (4.3%) progressed to invasive carcinoma after treatment 31 patients (67.4%) achieved disease control with in-office procedures alone Patients who failed treatment had a statistically significantly shorter period between treatments than responders (median, 2.3 mo vs 8.9 mo)	Biopsy ruled out invasive carcinoma before treatment initiation Patients underwent a median of 2 (range, 1–6) procedures at median intervals of 7.6 mo
Vascular lesions	Sheu et al,[9] 2012	3 lesions showed a reduction in mean lesion size at follow-up (4.10 pixels from 9.98 pixels)	

Vocal fold polyps	Sridharan et al,[25] 2014	Statistically significant reduction in VHI-10 scores before and after treatment (mean, 19.7 pretreatment to 9.7 at first follow-up, to 8.3 at second follow-up) for 31 patients undergoing in-office KTP laser procedures for vascular and nonvascular polyps Improvements in noise-to-harmonic ratio and speaking fundamental frequency in male and female patients	In the operating room, lesions were excised with "cold knife" technique In the office setting, polyps were treated with the KTP laser to produce a KTP type 2 effect, and the lesion was then removed with biopsy forceps
	Wang et al,[45] 2015	Compared outcomes of excision of vocal fold polyps via microlaryngoscopy under general anesthesia with in-office KTP laser treatment and polypectomy Patients who underwent in-office treatment reported higher subjective voice quality than those managed in the operating room at 2 wk follow-up No significant differences between the 2 groups with respect to objective (videostroboscopy, perceptual voice quality, and acoustic measures) and subjective (self-rated visual analog score, VHI-10 score) outcome measures at 6 wk Authors concluded that although both treatment options are effective, patients who underwent in-office management had more rapid improvement in symptoms	
Laryngeal granulomas	Mascarella & Young,[46] 2016	Base of vocal process granuloma cauterized with KTP laser, and the lesion was removed with biopsy forceps transnasally No recurrence at 1.5 y	Case report
	Dominguez et al,[47] 2017	26 patients underwent 43 in-office KTP laser procedures for laryngeal granulomas Decrease in lesion size in 96.2% of cases, and complete resolution of the granuloma in 73.1% More than half the cohort (53.8%) had complete resolution of their granuloma after a single treatment	Etiologies of the granulomas were noniatrogenic (laryngopharyngeal reflux, cough), vocal fold surgery (postcordotomy, postexcision of Teflon granuloma), and intubation

(continued on next page)

Table 2
(continued)

Lesion/Pathology	Authors/Year	Outcomes	Other Details
Reinke edema	Pitman et al,[48] 2012	7 patients with Reinke edema underwent in-office KTP laser treatment Intact mucosal wave in all patients post-treatment, decrease in median VHI-10 score (37–26), reduction in GRBAS score, and improvements in acoustic parameters (maximum phonation time and fundamental frequency)	Laser settings were 35 W, 15 ms pulse width
	Young et al,[49] 2015	Treatment of Reinke edema with in-office KTP laser procedures and microlaryngeal procedures in the operating room 9 patients, 10 treatments total VHI-10 scores decreased by a mean of 8.3 Treatment with type 1 or 2 effect and <200 J of energy yielded the most favorable voice outcomes (mean change in VHI-10 score of −7.2 for type 1 and −12 for type 2)	Laser settings were 15–35 W, 15 ms pulse width, 2 pps Average of 157 J administered over an average of 0.37 s of laser deployment Tissue effects induced ranged from KTP type 1–3
Other miscellaneous benign lesions	Mallur et al,[24] 2014	47 in-office KTP laser procedures for nonpapilloma laryngeal lesions: hemorrhagic polyps (23), nonhemorrhagic polyps (7), vocal process granulomas (7), Reinke edema (5), vocal fold cyst (1), pseudocyst (1), leukoplakia (1), squamous cell carcinoma in situ (1), vocal fold hemorrhage (1) Statistically significant reduction in lesion size 1 mo after treatment for all lesions except polyps When comparing the smallest lesion size during the 1-y follow-up period with the pretreatment size, a statistically significant decrease was seen for all lesions except Reinke edema	

Sheu et al,[9] 2012	Statistically significant reduction in lesion size across all diagnoses at initial and long-term follow up: vocal fold polyps (24), hemorrhagic polyps (13), granulomas (13), Reinke edema (8), vocal fold cyst (2), vocal fold scar (1), and amyloidosis (1) Within specific lesion categories, statistically significant reductions in lesion size for nonhemorrhagic and hemorrhagic polyps, granulomas, and Reinke edema Glottic closure and mucosal wave were either improved or unchanged in 92% and 95% of patients on videostroboscopy
Helman & Pitman,[50] 2017	4 patients with laryngeal and vallecular mucoceles Mucocele devascularized with KTP laser, then marsupialized with cup forceps No recurrence at follow-up of 6–12 mo

Abbreviations: GRBAS, grade of hoarseness, roughness, breathiness, asthenia, and strain; pps, pulses per second; VHI, voice handicap index.

Recurrent Respiratory Papillomatosis

RRP was one of the first laryngeal pathologies to be treated with in-office KTP laser procedures.[7] The KTP laser has also been combined with intralesional bevacizumab (Avastin) injection for the treatment of RRP.[37] These studies are detailed in **Table 2**. One concern regarding in-office laser procedures for management of RRP is the possible transmission of the human papilloma virus (HPV), two strains of which (HPV6 and HPV11) have been shown to be the most common causes of RPP.[38,39] Two studies have shown possible transfer of the virus from the patient to the surgeon.[40,41] A study by Dodhia and colleagues,[42] however, found no detectable HPV on sterilized or unsterilized KTP laser fibers that had been used for the treatment of RRP. These findings suggest that the virus is unlikely to be transferred from patients to the surgeon or other staff, especially if proper personal protective equipment is used and proper sterilization practices are followed.

Leukoplakia/Dysplasia

Treatment of keratosis with dysplasia was also described in the initial study on in-office KTP laser procedures by Zeitels and colleagues[7] in 2006. Outcomes in the management of leukoplakia with in-office KTP laser procedures were also detailed in the multi-institutional study by Sheu and colleagues[9] in 2012. Further support of the efficacy of serial in-office laser procedures for the management of leukoplakia was reported by Koss and colleagues[43] in 2017. These studies are listed in **Table 2**. Although leukoplakia is clearly amenable to in-office laser treatment, it is important to be mindful that these lesions are at risk for malignant transformation,[44] and biopsy should be performed at initial presentation and again if disease burden worsens despite treatment.

Vascular Lesions

Vascular lesions are ideal targets for the KTP laser, with its 532-nm wavelength being very close to the absorbance peaks of oxyhemoglobin (approximately 541 nm).[7] Zeitels and colleagues[8] first described the use of the KTP laser via direct microlaryngoscopy for treatment of vocal fold ectasias and varices in singers. The PDL laser was also used for some patients included in the study, and the authors concluded that although both modalities are safe and effective, the PDL laser carried a higher risk of vessel wall rupture. Treatment outcomes of in-office KTP laser treatment of vascular lesions were reported in the 2012 multi-institutional study by Sheu and colleagues[9] (see **Table 2**).

Miscellaneous Benign Lesions

In-office KTP laser procedures have been used to treat a variety of additional benign laryngeal lesions, including vocal fold polyps,[25,45] laryngeal granulomas,[46,47] and Reinke edema.[48,49] Details and outcomes of these studies are included in **Table 2**. Studies by Mallur and colleagues[24] and Sheu and colleagues[9] describe outcomes of in-office KTP laser treatment of a variety of benign lesions (see **Table 2**). The use of the KTP laser to manage laryngeal and vallecular mucoceles in the office setting was also recently described (see **Table 2**).[50]

There is limited information in the existing literature regarding the use of the KTP laser for vocal fold scar in the office setting. The previously mentioned multi-institutional study of KTP laser treatment of benign laryngeal lesions included only one patient with vocal fold scar, whose lesion did not decrease in size on follow-up examination.[9] Animal studies do show promise, however, with KTP laser treatment being shown to increase inflammatory gene expression and matrix metalloproteinase gene expression in a rat model of vocal fold injury.[51] Similar findings were demonstrated in a rabbit model of vocal fold scar.[52] Although these studies are encouraging, further study is necessary to determine the effectiveness of the KTP laser in the treatment of vocal fold scar.

CODING, BILLING, AND REIMBURSEMENT

From an early stage, the potential cost savings of in-office laryngeal procedures have been apparent. Studies have shown a cost savings of more than $5000 per case when procedures are performed in the office setting rather than the operating room.[11,53] Although there were clear benefits to patients as far as decreased cost because operating room and anesthesia charges were avoided, typically an unlisted code would be used for the procedure and reimbursement was variable. A study by Kuo and Halum[54] in 2012 demonstrated that reimbursement for in-office procedures did not cover costs associated with equipment, staff, and supplies, resulting in a financial loss of more than $500 per case. Performance of awake laser laryngeal surgery in a surgery center or endoscopy suite became a popular option, because hospitals and surgery centers may bill and be reimbursed for all staff, supplies, anesthetic, and operative time necessary for the procedure. Hillel and colleagues[55] compared the costs, charges, and reimbursements of performing awake laryngeal procedures in an endoscopy suite with performing similar procedures under general anesthesia in the operating room. The authors found that hospital expenses were significantly less when procedures were performed in the endoscopy suite. Because reimbursement was similar for the two settings, net balance of reimbursement minus expenses was greater for procedures performed in the endoscopy suite. In 2017, a specific Current Procedural Terminology code was developed for awake laser laryngeal procedures: 31,572 (laryngoscopy, flexible; with ablation or destruction of lesions with fiber-based laser, unilateral). A 50 modifier may be added for bilateral lesions. There is also now greater reimbursement when the procedure is performed in the nonfacility setting,[56] which may result in increased performance of these procedures in the office setting.

FUTURE ENDEAVORS

Over the last decade, the indications for in-office KTP laser laryngeal procedures have expanded dramatically, with new applications continuing to emerge in the literature. Unfortunately, the Aura XP KTP laser system is no longer in production, although the technology may be licensed to another company to manufacture new units in the future. Presumably, the systems will continue to be available for rent through mobile surgical supply companies, so surgeons who wish to expand their practices to include this modality will still have a means to do so. There may potentially be an increase in the use of other lasers in the office setting, such as CO_2 and PDL, if availability of the KTP laser decreases. The CO_2 laser (wavelength 10,600 nm), although originally only able to be operated via mirror-reflected line of sight delivery, is now deliverable via a fiber that may be passed through the working channel of a laryngoscope.[57–60] The thulium laser (wavelength 2013 nm) is similar to the CO_2 laser in that its chromophore is also water. Its coagulation capabilities are superior, however, leading to better hemostasis. It is delivered through a glass fiber that may be passed via the working channel of a laryngoscope, and can be used in contact and noncontact modes.[61] Despite the discontinuance of production of the KTP laser, the applications of in-office laryngeal procedures are likely to continue to increase.

SUMMARY

Advances in technology have led to the expansion of in-office procedures in laryngology, with laryngeal surgery now widely performed in the office setting. Patient preference and changes in coding and reimbursement have supported this trend. The indications for KTP laser laryngeal surgery have become numerous over the last several years, and there is strong support for this modality's safety and efficacy in the literature.

SUPPLEMENTARY DATA

Supplementary data related to this article can be found online at https://doi.org/10.1016/j.otc.2019.02.011.

REFERENCES

1. Simpson CB, Amin MR, Postma GN. Topical anesthesia of the airway and esophagus. Ear Nose Throat J 2004;83(7 Suppl 2):2–5.
2. Simpson CB, Amin MR. Office-based procedures for the voice. Ear Nose Throat J 2004;83(7 Suppl 2):6–9.
4. Carruth JA. The role of lasers in otolaryngology. World J Surg 1983;7(6):719–24.
3. Rosen CA, Amin MR, Sulica L, et al. Advances in office-based diagnosis and treatment in laryngology. Laryngoscope 2009;119(Suppl 2):S185–212.
5. Fried MP. Recent advances in laser otolaryngology. Keio J Med 1993;42(4):171–3.
6. Zeitels SM, Franco RA Jr, Dailey SH, et al. Office-based treatment of glottal dysplasia and papillomatosis with the 585-nm pulsed dye laser and local anesthesia. Ann Otol Rhinol Laryngol 2004;113:265–76.
7. Zeitels SM, Akst LM, Burns JA, et al. Office-based 532-nm pulsed KTP laser treatment of glottal papillomatosis and dysplasia. Ann Otol Rhinol Laryngol 2006;115(9):679–85.
8. Zeitels SM, Akst LM, Burns JA, et al. Pulsed angiolytic laser treatment of ectasias and varices in singers. Ann Otol Rhinol Laryngol 2006;115(8):571–80.
9. Sheu M, Sridharan S, Kuhn M, et al. Multi-institutional experience with the in-office potassium titanyl phosphate laser for laryngeal lesions. J Voice 2012;26(6):806–10.
10. Rees CJ, Halum SL, Wijewickrama C, et al. Patient tolerance of in-office pulsed dye laser treatment to the upper aerodigestive tract. Otolaryngol Head Neck Surg 2006;134:1023–7.
11. Halum SL, Moberly AC. Patient tolerance of the flexible CO2 laser for office-based laryngeal surgery. J Voice 2010;24:750–4.
12. Young VN, Smith LJ, Sulica L, et al. Patient tolerance of awake, in-office laryngeal procedures: a multi-institutional perspective. Laryngoscope 2012;122(2):315–21.
13. Anderson J, Bensoussan Y, Townsley R, et al. In-office endoscopic laryngeal laser procedures: a patient safety initiative. Otolaryngol Head Neck Surg 2018;159(1):136–42.
14. Yung KC, Courey MS. The effect of office-based flexible endoscopic surgery on hemodynamic stability. Laryngoscope 2010;120(11):2231–6.
15. Morrison MP, O'Rourke A, Dion GR, et al. Hemodynamic changes during otolaryngological office-based flexible endoscopic procedures. Ann Otol Rhinol Laryngol 2012;121(11):714–8.

16. Tierney WS, Chota RL, Benninger MS, et al. Hemodynamic parameters during laryngoscopic procedures in the office and in the operating room. Otolaryngol Head Neck Surg 2016;155(3):466–72.

17. Madden LL, Ward J, Ward A, et al. A cardiovascular prescreening protocol for unmonitored in-office laryngology procedures. Laryngoscope 2017;127(8):1845–9.

18. Wang SX, Simpson CB. Anesthesia for office procedures. Otolaryngol Clin North Am 2013;46(1):13–9.

19. McCaughey W. Adverse effects of local anaesthetics. Drug Saf 1992;7:178–89.

20. Fritz MA, Peng R, Born H, et al. The safety of antithrombotic therapy during in-office laryngeal procedures-a preliminary study. J Voice 2015;29(6):768–71.

21. Hogikyan ND. Transnasal endoscopic examination of the subglottis and trachea using topical anesthesia in the otolaryngology clinic. Laryngoscope 1999; 109(7 Pt 1):1170–3.

22. Bastian RW, Riggs LC. Role of sensation in swallowing function. Laryngoscope 1999;109(12):1974–7.

23. Adriani J, Campbell D. Fatalities following topical application of local anaesthetics to mucous membranes. JAMA 1956;162:1527–30.

24. Mallur PS, Johns MM 3rd, Amin MR, et al. Proposed classification system for reporting 532-nm pulsed potassium titanyl phosphate laser treatment effects on vocal fold lesions. Laryngoscope 2014;124(5):1170–5.

25. Sridharan S, Achlatis R, Ruiz R, et al. Patient-based outcomes of in-office KTP ablation of vocal fold polyps. Laryngoscope 2014;124:1176–9.

26. Postma GN, Goins MR, Koufman JA. Office-based laser procedures for the upper aerodigestive tract: emerging technology. Ear Nose Throat J 2004;83(7 Suppl 2): 22–4.

27. Bové MJ, Jabbour N, Krishna P, et al. Operating room versus office-based injection laryngoplasty: a comparative analysis of reimbursement. Laryngoscope 2007;117:226–30.

28. Postma GN, Cohen JT, Belafsky PC, et al. Transnasal esophagoscopy: revisited (over 700 consecutive cases). Laryngoscope 2005;115(2):321–3.

29. Koufman JA, Rees CJ, Frazier WD, et al. Office-based laryngeal laser surgery: a review of 443 cases using three wavelengths. Otolaryngol Head Neck Surg 2007; 137:146–51.

30. Del Signore AG, Shah RN, Gupta N, et al. Complications and failures of office-based endoscopic angiolytic laser surgery treatment. J Voice 2016;30(6):744–50.

31. Berde CB, Strichartz GR. Local anesthetics. In: Miller RD, Eriksson LI, Fleisher LA, et al, editors. Miller's anesthesia. 7th edition. Churchill, Livingstone Elsevier; 2009. p. 913–40.

32. Neal JM, Bernards CM, Butterworth JF 4th, et al. ASRA practice advisory on local anesthetic systemic toxicity. Reg Anesth Pain Med 2010;35(2):152–61.

33. Kwok S, Fischer JL, Rogers JD. Benzocaine and lidocaine induced methemoglobinemia after bronchoscopy: a case report. J Med Case Rep 2008;2:16.

34. Day AT, Rivera E, Farlow JL, et al. Surgical fires in otolaryngology: a systematic and narrative review. Otolaryngol Head Neck Surg 2018;158(4):598–616.

35. Yardley IE, Donaldson LJ. Surgical fires, a clear and present danger. Surgeon 2010;8:87–92.

36. Association of Surgical Technologists Standards of Practice for Laser Safety. Available at: http://www.cspsteam.org/7-fire-safety/. Accessed July 15, 2018.

37. Zeitels SM, Barbu AM, Landau-Zemer T, et al. Local injection of bevacizumab (Avastin) and angiolytic KTP laser treatment of recurrent respiratory

papillomatosis of the vocal folds: a prospective study. Ann Otol Rhinol Laryngol 2011;120(10):627–34.

38. De Villiers E-M, Fauquet C, Broker TR, et al. Classification of papillomaviruses. Virology 2004;324:17–27.

39. Dickens P, Srivastava G, Loke SL, et al. Human papillomavirus 6, 11, and 16 in laryngeal papillomas. J Pathol 1991;165:243–6.

40. Manson LT, Damrose EJ. Does exposure to laser plume place the surgeon at high risk for acquiring clinical human papillomavirus infection? Laryngoscope 2013; 123:1319–20.

41. Hallmo P, Naess O. Laryngeal papillomatosis with human papillomavirus DNA contracted by a laser surgeon. Eur Arch Otorhinolaryngol 1991;248:425–7.

42. Dodhia S, Baxter PC, Ye F, et al. Investigation of the presence of HPV on KTP laser fibers following KTP laser treatment of papilloma. Laryngoscope 2018; 128(4):926–8.

43. Koss SL, Baxter P, Panossian H, et al. Serial in-office laser treatment of vocal fold leukoplakia: disease control and voice outcomes. Laryngoscope 2017;127(7): 1644–51.

44. Isenberg JS, Crozier DL, Dailey SH. Institutional and comprehensive review of laryngeal leukoplakia. Ann Otol Rhinol Laryngol 2008;117:74–9.

45. Wang CT, Liao LJ, Huang TW, et al. Comparison of treatment outcomes of trans-nasal vocal fold polypectomy versus microlaryngoscopic surgery. Laryngoscope 2015;125(5):1155–60.

46. Mascarella MA, Young J. In-office excision en masse of a vocal process granu-loma using the potassium-titanyl-phosphate laser. J Voice 2016;30(1):93–5.

47. Dominguez LM, Brown RJ, Simpson CB. Treatment outcomes of in-office KTP ablation of vocal fold granulomas. Ann Otol Rhinol Laryngol 2017;126(12): 829–34.

48. Pitman MJ, Lebowitz-Cooper A, Iacob C, et al. Effect of the 532nm pulsed KTP laser in the treatment of Reinke's edema. Laryngoscope 2012;122(12):2786–92.

49. Young VN, Mallur PS, Wong AW, et al. Analysis of potassium titanyl phosphate laser settings and voice outcomes in the treatment of Reinke's edema. Ann Otol Rhinol Laryngol 2015;124(3):216–20.

50. Helman SN, Pitman MJ. Office-based 532-nanometer pulsed potassium-titanyl-phosphate laser for marsupialization of laryngeal and vallecular mucoceles. Laryngoscope 2017;127(5):1116–8.

51. Sheu M, Sridharan S, Paul B, et al. The utility of the potassium titanyl phosphate laser in modulating vocal fold scar in a rat model. Laryngoscope 2013;123(9): 2189–94.

52. Zhang J, Zhen R, Wei C. Potassium titanyl phosphate laser-induced inflammatory response and extracellular matrix turnover in rabbit vocal fold scar. Eur Arch Oto-rhinolaryngol 2018;275(6):1525–32.

53. Rees CJ, Postma GN, Koufman JA. Cost savings of unsedated office-based laser surgery for laryngeal papillomas. Ann Otol Rhinol Laryngol 2007;116:45–8.

54. Kuo CY, Halum SL. Office-based laser surgery of the larynx: cost-effective treat-ment at the office's expense. Otolaryngol Head Neck Surg 2012;146(5):769–73.

55. Hillel AT, Ochsner MC, Johns MM 3rd, et al. A cost and time analysis of laryn-gology procedures in the endoscopy suite versus the operating room. Laryngo-scope 2016;126(6):1385–9.

56. Centers for Medicare and Medicaid Services. Available at: www.cms.gov. Ac-cessed July 15, 2018.

57. Devaiah AK, Shapshay SM, Desai U, et al. Surgical utility of a new carbon dioxide laser fiber: functional and histological study. Laryngoscope 2005;115:1463–8.

58. Zeitels SM, Kobler JB, Heaton JT, et al. Carbon dioxide laser fiber for laryngeal cancer surgery. Ann Otol Rhinol Laryngol 2006;115:535–41.

59. Shurgalin M, Anastassiou C. A new modality for minimally invasive CO_2 laser surgery: flexible hollow-core photonic bandgap fibers. Biomed Instrum Technol 2008;42:318–25.

60. Wang Z, Chocat N. Fiber-optic technologies in laser-based therapeutics: threads for a cure. Curr Pharm Biotechnol 2010;11:384–97.

61. Zeitels SM, Burns JA, Akst LM, et al. Office-based and microlaryngeal applications of a fiber-based thulium laser. Ann Otol Rhinol Laryngol 2006;115:891–6.

In-Office Ultrasonographic Evaluation of Neck Masses/ Thyroid Nodules

Cristian M. Slough, MD[a], Dipti Kamani, MD[b],
Gregory W. Randolph, MD, FACS, FACE[b,c],*

KEYWORDS

- Ultrasound • Head and neck ultrasound • Office-based ultrasound
- Thyroid ultrasound • Evaluation of neck nodes • Fine-needle aspiration

KEY POINTS

- Office-based ultrasonography is increasingly becoming an integral part of in-office evaluation in otolaryngology head and neck surgery practice.
- A thorough knowledge of complex head and neck anatomy, and ultrasonographic appearance of normal and abnormal pathology are key for performing/interpreting office-based head and neck ultrasonographic examination.
- A focused but systematic approach allows for efficient and effective office-based head and neck ultrasonographic examination.
- Ultrasound-guided fine-needle aspiration is an integral part of clinician-performed ultrasonography because it allows cytologic diagnosis of suspicious lesions.
- Training in the form of certification or accreditation is recommended for clinicians planning to perform office-based head and neck ultrasonography.

INTRODUCTION

Although ultrasonography of the head and neck has been performed for decades, recent advances in technology and miniaturization have allowed office-based ultrasonography to become not only a reality but indeed a necessity for most head and neck surgeons. Originally performed by radiologists, improved accessibility and appropriate training for otolaryngologists, surgeons, and emergency room providers have

Disclosure: The authors have nothing to disclose.
[a] Willamette Valley Ear, Nose, & Throat, Willamette Valley Medical Center, 2700 SE Stratus Ave, McMinnville, OR 97128, USA; [b] Division of Thyroid and Parathyroid Surgery, Department of Otolaryngology, Massachusetts Eye and Ear, Harvard Medical School, 243, Charles Street, Boston, MA 02114, USA; [c] Division of Surgical Oncology, Endocrine Surgery Service, Department of Surgery, Massachusetts General Hospital, Harvard Medical School, Boston, MA, USA
* Corresponding author. 243 Charles Street, Boston, MA 02114.
E-mail address: gregory_randolph@meei.harvard.edu

expanded the application of this imaging modality. The main advantage of the treating physician/provider performing the ultrasonographic examination is the enhancement of the clinician's ability to examine the patient dynamically, with the patient's differential diagnosis coupled with the knowledge of the head and neck anatomy. Routine office-based ultrasonography is an important extension of the history/physical examination and maximizes efficiency by aiding in prompt diagnosis. The ultrasonographic examination is integral to preoperative planning and to long-term follow-up. A thorough knowledge of the complex anatomy of the head and neck region as well as familiarity with the ultrasonographic appearance of normal structures and abnormal pathology are essential for performing and interpreting head and neck ultrasonography.

However, ultrasonographic examinations can be time consuming, the equipment can be expensive, and at times interpretation may be limited by the patient's anatomy, limited neck mobility, tolerance of positioning, and objection by radiology colleagues of its use by the surgeon. These obstacles can be overcome by open conversations among the medical staff, inclusion of a mechanism to share or maintain the images, and a comprehensive report for future follow-up assessment beyond the provider's clinic.[1]

HEAD AND NECK ULTRASONOGRAPHY: TECHNIQUE AND A SYSTEMATIC APPROACH

The key element to a successful, efficient, and comprehensive head and neck ultrasonography is a consistently systematic protocol to ensure that all structures of the neck from clavicle to mandible are accurately evaluated. An ultrasonographic appreciation of the echogenic characteristics of various normal tissue types in the head and neck allows the identification of what is normal and what is pathologic. The neck is imaged using a high-frequency linear transducer, at 8 to 15 MHz, depending on the thickness of the patient's neck, but greater than 7.5 MHz, with color Doppler capability. Most transducers have a notch or indicator on one side. By convention, this is oriented toward the patient's right side or superiorly, ensuring the correct orientation of the ultrasonographic image, with the left side of the image representing the patient's right side on the transverse view, and cephalad on the sagittal view.

A targeted limited approach is often applied to head and neck ultrasonography, but we prefer a focused but systematic approach[2] (**Fig. 1**). This allows the clinician to focus on the concerned region while still effectively and efficiently performing the rest of the head and neck examination. A systematic approach for office-based head and neck ultrasonography is key to reproducibility, adequate evaluation of underlying pathology, and to avoid the common pitfall of omission. The examination should include visceral structures, the central and lateral compartment of the neck in both longitudinal and transverse planes, with special attention to the thyroid gland, trachea, esophagus, and associated nodal basins. It is important to describe the precise location, to note important features for cancer management and staging, and to review "check locations." Check locations are locations to "check" when certain pathology is identified such as the thyroid gland in a case of thyroglossal duct cyst.[3]

ULTRASONOGRAPHIC APPEARANCE OF NORMAL NECK STRUCTURES

An ultrasonographic appreciation of the echogenic characteristics of various normal head and neck tissue types facilitates the identification of abnormal pathology. The strong echogenicity of the cervical fascia, the hypoechoic musculature in contrast to the hyperechoic adipose tissue allows division of the neck sonographically into

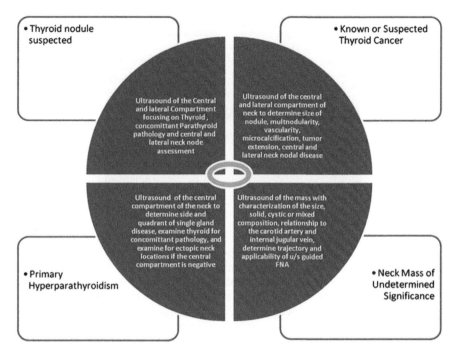

Fig. 1. Systematic, focused approach to neck ultrasonography. (*From* Bumpous JM, Randolph GW. The expanding utility of office-based ultrasound for the head and neck surgeon. Otolaryngol Clin North Am 2010;43(6):1203–8, vi; with permission.)

its well-recognized triangles. The salivary glands appear homogeneous and slightly hyperechoic compared with surrounding muscle (**Fig. 2**). Intraglandular ducts may be identified as small linear hyperechoic lines, and salivary ducts sometimes appear as tubular structures that are best seen when pathologically dilated. The parotid gland can have intraparotid lymph nodes, whereas the submandibular gland does not. It is important to be aware of Küttner lymph nodes, often mistaken for submandibular pathology, having a close relationship to the submandibular gland posteriorly and adjacent to the parotid gland (**Fig. 3**). The retromandibular vein, just posterior to the submandibular gland, is a useful landmark to delineate the parotid space from the submandibular space.[4]

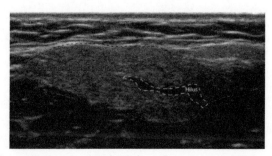

Fig. 2. Normal submandibular gland with its classic homogeneous appearance while slightly hyperechoic compared with surrounding muscle.

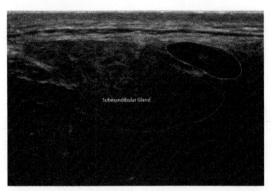

Fig. 3. Küttner lymph node (*yellow dotted line*) adjacent to the submandibular gland (*red dotted line*). The normal fatty hilum of the lymph node can be seen.

The arteries are identified as anechoic pulsatile structures, and similar structures with compressibility are identified as veins. Carotid bifurcation, visualized by tracing the carotid artery superiorly is a useful landmark. Color Doppler aids in confirmation of these structures (**Fig. 4**). Lymph nodes are often visualized along the course of these major vessels as circular or ovoid structures with echogenic fatty hilum; color Doppler can show their afferent and efferent lymphatics (**Fig. 5**). Lymph nodes can also be seen in the other neck triangles, and their characteristic appearance allows easy identification.[5]

The thyroid gland is easily identified by its characteristic location, shape, and homogeneous and hyperechoic parenchymal appearance. It is invested by fascia with a similar echogenic appearance to the fascia around the musculature. Normal parathyroid glands are rarely visible sonographically and are generally only visible when involved in a pathologic process.

The trachea lies posterior to the thyroid, and the common carotid arteries border the gland laterally on each side. The trachea has a characteristic appearance on ultrasonography with the complete cricoid ring superiorly and the cartilaginous tracheal rings inferiorly. The esophagus is typically seen inferiorly, deep to the left thyroid lobe, as concentric circles of varying echogenicity (**Fig. 6**). Swallowing instantaneously broadens the esophagus, and hyperechoic saliva mixed with air can be seen in transit

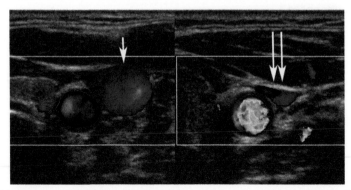

Fig. 4. Side-by-side comparison of the carotid artery and internal jugular vein demonstrating the resting state of the vein (*single arrow*) versus compressed (*double arrows*).

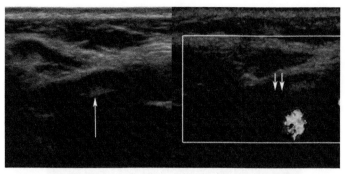

Fig. 5. Normal lymph node with a fatty hilum (*single arrow*) and evidence of blood flow on color Doppler (*double arrow*).

in the esophageal lumen, further aiding its identification.[6] Ultrasonographically, the larynx is composed of echogenic cartilaginous structures in contrast to its hypoechoic intrinsic musculature, lined by the hyperechoic mucosa and anechoic internal airway[5] (**Fig. 7**).

ULTRASONOGRAPHIC EVALUATION OF THE THYROID GLAND

Ultrasonography is the single most-valuable imaging modality in the evaluation of the thyroid gland.[7] The location, signature echogenicity, and distinct sonographic features of different thyroid pathologies make ultrasonography a powerful tool for assessment in the thyroid gland, often providing greater detail than other imaging modalities.[8] Thyroid ultrasonographic examinations are mainly performed for the evaluation of thyroid nodules, many incidentally discovered (**Fig. 8**). Caution should be exercised for using thyroid ultrasonography as a screening tool for the detection of nodules given a prevalence rate as high as 50%.[9] Ultrasonography of the thyroid achieves several goals, including the confirmation of a thyroid nodule, depiction of its size, location, identification of benign versus suspicious features, evaluation for cervical lymphadenopathy, and allowing ultrasound-guided fine-needle aspiration (USgFNA).

Familiarity with the specific ultrasonographic features that are suggestive of malignancy, namely hypoechogenicity, irregular or blurred margins, microcalcifications,

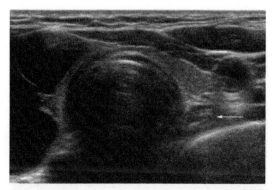

Fig. 6. Esophagus in its usual position on the left side posterior to the left thyroid lobe with its concentric ring appearance (*single arrow*) not to be confused with a thyroid nodule.

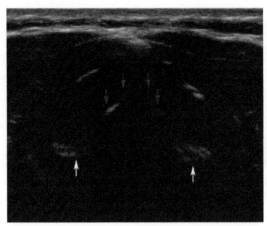

Fig. 7. Normal appearance of the larynx with hypoechoic intrinsic musculature, lined by the hyperechoic mucosa (*red arrows*), anechoic internal airway, and hyperechoic arytenoids (*white arrows*).

taller than wider shape, and vascular signals, is important.[10] A hypoechoic nodule has a higher propensity for malignancy compared with an iso/hyperechoic nodule.[10,11] Solid nodules are suggestive of malignancy, whereas increasingly cystic nodules are more likely benign, and completely cystic nodules are certainly benign.[12] Irregular or blurred margins are associated with malignancy.[11] Fixation of the gland further suggests malignancy, with invasion of the surrounding tissue.[8] Some authors have questioned the predictive value of the "taller than wider" nodular shape, with some studies suggesting that spherical nodules have a higher incidence of malignancy.[8] The vascular pattern of the nodule has been correlated with risk of malignancy and increases as intranodular blood flow becomes more dominant.[13] Microcalcifications within the nodule increase the risk of malignancy of the nodule and should prompt fine-needle aspiration (FNA) in most cases[10,11,14] (**Fig. 9**).

The use of ultrasound guidance has improved overall sensitivity (97.2%–100%), specificity (50%–70.9%) and increased adequacy of sampling (92.9%–96.5%) and, thereby, improved global diagnostic accuracy (75.9%–80%) in the thyroid nodule

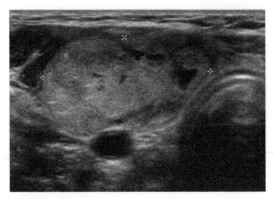

Fig. 8. Right thyroid lobe nodule.

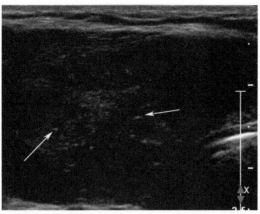

Fig. 9. Thyroid nodule with microcalcifications (*white arrows*). Used with permission from the American College of Radiology.

assessment compared with palpation-guided FNA.[15,16] This is particularly true for smaller nonpalpable nodules, mixed solid and cystic nodules, and for repeat FNA of nondiagnostic nodules.[7,16]

There are 3 main published and validated ultrasonography classification criteria for stratifying malignancy risk and determining the need for FNA.[7,9,17] All thyroid nodule management guidelines recommend FNA by considering the above characteristics with nodule size thresholds. These classification systems also improve communication among clinicians and help standardize clinical practice.

The revised American Thyroid Association (ATA) proposed 5 levels of risk stratification: benign, very low, low, intermediate, and high suspicion for malignancy.[7] Subsequently, the American Association of Clinical Endocrinologists (AACE), American College of Endocrinology (ACE), and Associazione Medici Endocrinologi (AME) guideline proposed 3 risk categories: low (class 1), intermediate (class 2), and high (class 3).[9] The American College of Radiology (ACR) has proposed the newest classification system, namely the Thyroid Imaging Reporting and Data System (TI-RADS). In the TI-RADS classification, based on the ultrasonographic features, the nodules are categorized as benign, minimally suspicious, moderately suspicious, or highly suspicious for malignancy. Points are given for all the ultrasonographic features (per lexicon category) of a nodule, with more suspicious features being awarded additional points and therefore lowering the size threshold for recommended biopsy of the nodule[17] **(Fig. 10)**.

One study comparing all 3 classifications systems found significant differences in the overall performance for the identification of high-risk cytology nodules, with ACR TI-RADS having the highest statistical concordance, similar to the AACE/ACE/ AME, but significantly higher than the ATA scheme. When considered separately, the AACE/ACE/AME highest-risk category provided the highest sensitivity (77%) but low specificity (63.5%), whereas the ATA and the ACR TI-RADS highest-risk categories provided high specificity (91.2% and 92.1%, respectively) but low sensitivity (41.6% and 41.7%, respectively). Furthermore, both the ATA and the AACE/ACE/ AME tools did not allow the classification of some nodules (up to 5% in ATA and 2.6% in the AACE/ACE/AME systems), whereas the ACR TI-RADS system allowed the classification of all nodules.[18] Of the unclassified nodules (2.6%–5%), only the ATA classification system missed a significant proportion (odds ratio = 7.2 compared

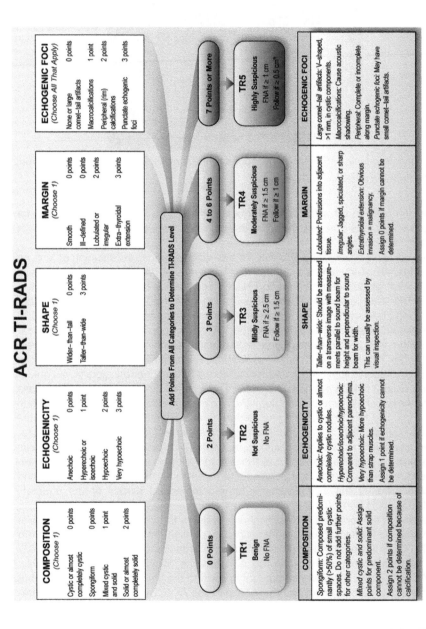

Fig. 10. ACR TI-RADS classification. [a] Refers to discussion of papillary carcinomas for 5–9-mm TR5 nodules. (*From* Tessler FN, Middleton WD, Grant EG, et al. ACR thyroid imaging, reporting and data system (TI-RADS): white paper of the ACR TI-RADS Committee. J Am Coll Radiol 2017;14(5):587–95; with permission.)

with 1.86 for the AACE/ACE/AME system) of nodules with a subsequent malignant cytology.[18]

Thyroid ultrasonography can also be used to detect Graves disease, thyroiditis, and subacute or de Quervain thyroiditis. The features of Graves disease include heterogeneous thyroid tissue with diffuse hypoechogenicity and hypervascularity, whereas those of Hashimoto thyroiditis include ill-defined hypoechoic areas separated by echogenic septa, with increased (early) or decreased (late) vascularity.[8] Subacute or de Quervain thyroiditis is more often a clinical diagnosis, but its characteristic ultrasonographic findings are ill-defined hypoechoic areas, without round or ovoid mass formation on multiple planes, and no vascular flow on color Doppler.[19]

Finally, ultrasonography is recommended for surveillance of cytologically benign thyroid nodules. The malignant transformation of benign thyroid nodules is rare but, given the 3% false-negative rate of FNA, continued surveillance is recommended. Both the ATA and the AACE/AME recommend 6- to 18-monthly follow-up of cytologically benign thyroid nodules with palpation if easily palpable, or with ultrasonography if not easily palpable.[7,9] Conversely, TI-RADS at times recommends that "no follow-up" is required, but do suggest that a patient or a provider's preferences may at times warrant deviation from the strict ACR TI-RADS guidelines. Patients with a strong personal or family history that increases the likelihood of cancer, or patients/providers who are highly concerned for other reasons, may recommend FNA or follow-up of nodules that are less than ACR TI-RADS size thresholds.[20] In our practice, we follow the ATA/AACE/AME-recommended guideline of 6- to 18-month follow-up, even for cytologically benign nodules or nodules that are deemed "no follow-up required" on TI-RADS.

Repeat FNA is recommended when there is evidence of nodule growth, defined as a volume change of greater than 50% or increase by greater than 20%, or greater than 2 mm in at least 2 dimensions in solid nodules or in the solid portion of a mixed cystic-solid nodule.[7,9]

Finally, important limitations of thyroid gland ultrasonography include its inability to assess substernal extent, airway invasion, and to identify definite pathology in a multinodular goiter.[21,22]

ULTRASONOGRAPHY OF NECK LYMPHATICS

Metastasis to cervical lymph nodes is common in thyroid carcinomas. The risk of disease recurrence, disease progression, and ultimately disease-specific mortality is related to completeness of surgical resection of the primary tumor and metastatic nodes, particularly for intermediate and high-risk patients with thyroid cancer.[23,24] Unrecognized metastatic lymph nodes are a common cause of persistent disease.[25] Therefore, nodal assessment is integral to thyroid nodule work-up, particularly when malignancy is suspected/diagnosed. Sonographic evaluation of neck nodes consists of 2 essential parts: grayscale and Doppler ultrasonography. Initial assessment evaluates the lymph node's size, shape, internal architecture, margins, the presence/absence of an echogenic hilus, cystic degeneration, and intranodal calcification. Doppler evaluation allows further assessment of the hilum, distribution of intranodal vessels, and vascular pattern of the lymph node.[8] Presence of microcalcifications, cystic degeneration, peripheral vascularity versus hilar vascularity, enlargement, a rounded shape versus ovoid, irregular or indistinct margins, or extracapsular extension suggest malignancy.[26] Notably, during lymph node size evaluation, the minimal axial diameter of the node is usually reported, because it is the most accurate dimension for predicting malignancy.[27] Reporting the location of abnormal lymph nodes using imaging-based nodal classification is helpful. Recently, Cunnane and colleagues[25] proposed a nodal classification that provides a simple, uniform, and reproducible basis for accurate communication of the nodal disease among multiple specialists (**Table 1**). It also assists in creating a radiographic map useful for intraoperative reference as well as for follow-up surveillance.

Preoperative ultrasonography for the central neck compartment with an intact thyroid gland is much less sensitive in revealing metastatic nodes, because they can be concealed by the thyroid gland.[28] Similarly, interpretation of preoperative FNA of these lymph nodes may also be questionable because of possible contamination by thyroid tissue. Nonetheless, the central compartment should be examined in all ultrasonographs and mapped preoperatively, but one should be cognizant that negative results on preoperative ultrasonography performed before thyroidectomy do not rule out metastatic central lymph nodes.

ULTRASONOGRAPHY OF THE PARATHYROID GLAND

Imaging for normal parathyroid glands is rarely used, because they are unidentifiable by virtue of their small size. However, adenomas enlarge the gland and hence can be localized on ultrasonography.[29] Ultrasonography effectively identifies and localizes abnormal parathyroid glands, mainly adenomas, but also carcinomas. Coupling the surgeon's knowledge of the embryology, anatomy, vascular supply, normal, and ectopic locations with real-time surgical planning allows the surgeon to visualize parathyroid adenomas in dynamic relation to nearby structures.[30,31] Ultrasonography can also evaluate multiglandular parathyroid disease.

Table 1
The imaging-based nodal classification

MEEI Symbols	Lymph Node Groups	Description
A	Right lateral neck	Inferior to the digastric muscle, posterior to submandibular gland, deep to the sternocleidomastoid muscle. This includes nodes that lie either anterior or posterior to the common carotid artery
B	Left lateral neck	Inferior to the digastric muscle, posterior to submandibular gland, deep to the sternocleidomastoid muscle. This includes nodes located either anterior or posterior to the common carotid artery
C	Right central neck	Nodes located medial to the common carotid artery, between it and the trachea
D	Left central neck	Nodes located medial to the common carotid artery, between it and the trachea
T	Pretracheal	Nodes located anterior to the trachea, between 10 and 2 on the clockface
L	Prelaryngeal	Nodes located anterior to the thyroid cartilage or the hyoid bone
E	Ectopic	Nodes located in sites outside typical neck regions. These ectopic sites include retropharyngeal, mediastinal, and axillary regions

From Cunnane M, Kyriazidis N, Kamani D, et al. A novel thyroid cancer nodal map classification system to facilitate nodal localization and surgical management: the A to D map. Laryngoscope 2017;127(10):2429–36; with permission.

Parathyroid adenomas are homogeneously hypoechoic in relation to the overlying thyroid gland and are often detected on grayscale alone. Smaller adenomas are usually oval/bean-shaped, but larger adenomas can be multilobulated. A side-by-side comparison of ultrasonographic images of parathyroid adenoma and normal cervical lymph node is depicted in **Fig. 11**. Doppler imaging can differentiate cervical lymph nodes from adenomas, because adenomas commonly show a characteristic extrathyroidal feeding vessel entering the parathyroid gland at one of the poles with a typical arc or rim vascularity versus the traditional hilar vessel.[29]

The accuracy of localization of ultrasonography for parathyroid adenomas can be limited by thick, obese neck, intrathyroidal lesions, multinodular disease, as well as by adenomas in ectopic locations behind bony or cartilaginous structures or structures containing air, such as the tracheoesophageal groove.[32] Ultrasonography performed by head and neck surgeons is reported to correctly predict surgical findings and localized disease in greater than 79% to 90% of cases.[30,31,33,34] Studies report that surgeon-performed, office-based, high-resolution ultrasonography is more accurate for preoperative localization of parathyroid adenomas than sestamibi Tc99m.[30,35]

The precise anatomic detail provided by ultrasonographic assessment facilitates successful focused parathyroidectomy and minimally invasive parathyroid surgeries in most patients.[34]

Bilateral, 4-gland explorations, used as an initial surgery for primary hyperparathyroidism, are reported to have greater than 95% success rate. Similar success rates are reported for focal explorations using preoperative localization with intraoperative parathyroid hormone measurement.[36,37]

Furthermore, office ultrasonography allows the surgeon to correlate ultrasonographic findings with additional studies such as sestamibi scan, computed tomography (CT), magentic resonance imaging, and, when indicated, the surgeon can also perform USgFNA with parathyroid hormone assay. Several studies report a high positive predictive value (100%) and specificity (100%) for parathyroid hormone washout.[38–40]

ULTRASONOGRAPHY OF THE SALIVARY GLANDS

Ultrasonography is not the preferred imaging modality for the salivary glands because of its inability to visualize the salivary glands completely, particularly the parotid gland, given the acoustic shadow of the mandible.

The most common pathologies of the salivary glands are inflammatory in nature, generally appearing on ultrasonography as enlargement of a gland that has lost

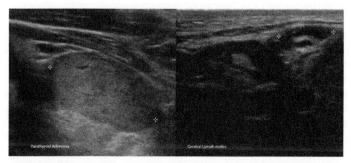

Fig. 11. Comparative figures of the sonographic appearance of normal cervical lymph nodes versus a parathyroid adenoma.

homogeneity, with Doppler showing increased blood flow. A hypoechoic or anechoic area with posterior acoustic enhancement and unclear borders in this setting may suggest the presence of an abscess.[41] Often, chronic sialoadenitis does not show gland enlargement or increased blood flow. Ultrasonographic features of sialolithiasis include hyperechoic lines/points with distal acoustic shadowing, which represent stones; visible dilated excretory ducts may be present in cases of duct occlusion.[42] Cysts within salivary glands are easily identified as hypoechoic lesions, whereas lymphoepithelial lesions in patients who are HIV positive may manifest as multiple cysts.[43]

Sonography of the salivary glands is useful to identify neoplasms, but diagnosis of benign versus malignant tumors is usually not possible.[42] However, certain ultrasonographic characteristics aid in this distinction. Calcifications, depth of the tumor from the surface, poorly defined border, irregular shape, and heterogenous echotexture correlate with malignant histology. In-office ultrasonography and USgFNA by a trained surgeon are an appropriate initial approach for evaluation of parotid lesions and can obviate additional imaging.[44,45]

ULTRASOUND-GUIDED BIOPSY AND CYTOPATHOLOGY

Ultrasound-guided fine-needle aspiration is an integral part of clinician-performed ultrasonography because it allows cytologic diagnosis of suspicious lesions. Ultrasound-guided fine-needle aspiration has been proven to be more efficient than conventional FNA, particularly for nodules located deep in the thyroid lobes, before cytologically nondiagnostic nodules, and for mixed solid cystic nodules.[46,47] Ultrasound-guided fine-needle aspiration performed by experienced surgeons has a high sensitivity (83.3%), specificity (98.8%), positive predictive value (97.0%), and negative predictive value (92.5%).[48] The rates of adequate samples obtained by USgFNA performed by surgeons newly trained in thyroid ultrasonography were similar to those obtained by experienced practitioners.[49]

Attention to technical details can improve cytologic results. Smaller needles (25 and 27 G) are superior to larger ones; a shorter "dwell time" (the time the needle is kept in the lesion) is often superior to longer dwell times, which introduce more blood; and rapid oscillations within the nodule (2 to 5 per second) are better than slow excursions.[8] Local anesthesia (1% lidocaine with 1:200,000 epinephrine), superficially to the skin, is generally recommended after the proposed USgFNA site is marked out, but before USgFNA. This improves patient tolerance of the USgFNA and reduces bruising after the procedure. However, care is taken not to infiltrate local anesthetic too deeply into the thyroid parenchyma so as not to affect sampling via dilution.

On-site cytopathology improves cytologic diagnosis of in-office USgFNA; cytopathologists have been consistently shown to enhance the USgFNA diagnosis with on-site assistance and training of the clinician performing the USgFNA.[50,51]

The complications of FNA include discomfort, hematoma, tracheal puncture, transient dysphagia, and a vasovagal reaction. The complication rate associated with FNA is low; a large study has reported a rate of 0.15%.[52] With careful visualization and avoidance of major vascular structures in the neck, USgFNA can safely be performed in patients who are anticoagulated and do not routinely need to stop their anticoagulation before USgFNA. Studies examining USgFNA in patients who are anticoagulated have not found that this factor increases the risk of complications, nor does it decrease the diagnostic yield.[53,54]

ADDITIONAL THERAPEUTIC APPLICATIONS OF HEAD AND NECK ULTRASONOGRAPHY

As the clinician sonographer becomes more familiar and comfortable with this imaging modality and performing USgFNA, ultrasonography becomes useful for other purposes in the clinic as an extension of a physician's clinical examination. It also becomes a useful adjunct to evaluate patients who previously may have required additional imaging modalities such as CT. The role of ultrasonography and the facets of its use are ever expanding as demonstrated by several studies lobbying for the use of head and neck ultrasonography in the office. Su and colleagues[55] report the use of office-based ultrasonography for injecting botulinum toxin to treat omohyoid syndrome with a good response lasting approximately 6 months. Ultrasound-guided sclerotherapy for certain benign nonthyroid cystic neck masses is promising as a potentially less-invasive management strategy.[56] Peritonsillar abscesses have been successfully identified using ultrasonography. Whereas an intraoral ultrasonographic probe is generally required, some have had success using a transcutaneous approach, obviating the need for CT imaging.[57,58] This approach is particularly useful for children, in whom ultrasonography has been shown to be reliable and highly correlative with surgical findings and clinical outcomes.[59,60] Some authors have advocated for ultrasound-guided drainage of abscesses, even deep abscesses. Good results have been obtained without recurrence or need for formal incision and drainage, and with a reduced hospital stay and cost savings overall.[61]

RECOMMENDED TRAINING, CERTIFICATION, AND ACCREDITATION

Training in the form of certification or accreditation is recommended for clinicians planning to perform office-based head and neck ultrasonography. There are several certification pathways for the clinician sonographer with courses offered by the American College of Surgeons, the AACE, and the Endocrine Society.

Most of these organizations provide an introductory course offering hands-on instruction in head and neck ultrasonography as well as USgFNA. Some of the courses require completion of an online course before attending the instructional course. The instructional portion is generally a 2-day course offered several times a year at multiple locations.

Ultrasonography accreditation is more complex than certification, but is valuable for those performing office-based head and neck ultrasonography routinely. Unlike certification, ultrasonography accreditation comprises all aspects of ultrasonography in clinical practice, including: clinician training and experience, ultrasonography protocols, ultrasonography machine maintenance and calibrations, and evaluation of actual case studies. There are 2 main pathways for accreditation, namely the American Institute of Ultrasound in Medicine (AIUM) in conjunction with the American Academy of Otolaryngology-Head and Neck Surgery (AAO-HNS) and the Endocrine Certification in Neck Ultrasound (ECNU). The ECNU comprises similar steps to accreditation as the AIUM/AAO-HNS route, but also includes a written Comprehensive Certification Examination as an initial step for accreditation. Some third-party payers require accreditation in ultrasonography as a condition for reimbursement.

CODING FOR OFFICE-BASED HEAD AND NECK ULTRASONOGRAPHY

Coding for head and neck ultrasonography can be complex and geographically dependent. Diagnostic ultrasonography of neck soft tissues include the use of Doppler codes with a Current Procedural Terminology code of 76536. If a USgFNA is performed, a code of 76942 is used for ultrasound needle guidance and 10022 for the actual USgFNA. A detailed and thorough review of the coding for head and neck ultrasonography can be found on the AACE Web site.

Coding and billing are dependent on documentation, and therefore storage of relevant images is a critical part of in-office ultrasonography and medicolegally prudent. Storage of in-office ultrasonographic images can be achieved by way of uploading to the electronic medical record, or, where available, uploading to the local picture archiving and communication system (PACS). Uploading to a PACS system, used by other local providers and radiologists, allows easier access and storage of the images, and permits easier transmission to other providers both locally and nationally. PACS also allows a formal report produced by the treating provider to be attached to the images for added correlation to the corresponding images.

SUMMARY

Office-based ultrasonography is increasingly becoming an integral part of an otolaryngology head and neck surgery practice. A thorough knowledge of the ultrasonic appearance of normal and abnormal pathology is key for performing/interpreting office-based head and neck ultrasonography. A methodical but systematic approach allows for efficient and effective office-based head and neck ultrasonography. Ultrasound-guided fine-needle aspiration is an integral part of clinician-performed ultrasonography, because it allows cytologic diagnosis of suspicious lesions. Office-based ultrasonography expands the otolaryngologist's armamentarium, enabling imaging and additional procedures in the office. Given the ease of using this imaging modality, and its accessibility, we highly recommend it.

REFERENCES

1. Symonds CJ, Seal P, Ghaznavi S, et al. Thyroid nodule ultrasound reports in routine clinical practice provide insufficient information to estimate risk of malignancy. Endocrine 2018;1–5. https://doi.org/10.1007/s12020-018-1634-0.
2. Bumpous JM, Randolph GW. The expanding utility of office-based ultrasound for the head and neck surgeon. Otolaryngol Clin North Am 2010;43(6):1203–8, vi.
3. Hoang JK, Vanka J, Ludwig BJ, et al. Evaluation of cervical lymph nodes in head and neck cancer with CT and MRI: tips, traps, and a systematic approach. AJR Am J Roentgenol 2013;200(1):W17–25.
4. Alyas F, Lewis K, Williams M, et al. Diseases of the submandibular gland as demonstrated using high resolution ultrasound. Br J Radiol 2005;78(928):362–9.
5. Klem C. Head and neck anatomy and ultrasound correlation. Otolaryngol Clin North Am 2010;43(6):1161–9. https://doi.org/10.1016/j.otc.2010.08.005, v.
6. Zhu S-Y, Liu R-C, Chen L-H, et al. Sonographic anatomy of the cervical esophagus. J Clin Ultrasound 2004;32(4):163–71. https://doi.org/10.1002/jcu.20017.
7. Haugen BR, Alexander EK, Bible KC, et al. 2015 American Thyroid Association Management guidelines for adult patients with thyroid nodules and differentiated thyroid cancer: the American Thyroid Association guidelines task force on thyroid nodules and differentiated thyroid cancer. Thyroid 2016;26(1):1–133.
8. Randolph G. Surgery of the thyroid and parathyroid glands. Philadelphia: Elsevier Health Sciences; 2012.
9. Gharib H, Papini E, Garber JR, et al. American Association of Clinical Endocrinologists, American College of Endocrinology, and Associazione Medici

Endocrinologi Medical guidelines for clinical practice for the diagnosis and management of thyroid nodules–2016 update. Endocr Pract 2016;22(5):622–39.

10. Kim E-K, Park CS, Chung WY, et al. New sonographic criteria for recommending fine-needle aspiration biopsy of nonpalpable solid nodules of the thyroid. AJR Am J Roentgenol 2002;178(3):687–91.

11. Cappelli C, Castellano M, Pirola I, et al. The predictive value of ultrasound findings in the management of thyroid nodules. QJM 2007;100(1):29–35.

12. Frates MC, Benson CB, Doubilet PM, et al. Prevalence and distribution of carcinoma in patients with solitary and multiple thyroid nodules on sonography. J Clin Endocrinol Metab 2006;91(9):3411–7.

13. Chammas MC, Gerhard R, De Oliveira IRS, et al. Thyroid nodules: evaluation with power Doppler and duplex Doppler ultrasound. Otolaryngol Head Neck Surg 2016;132(6):874–82.

14. Seiberling KA, Dutra JC, Grant T, et al. Role of intrathyroidal calcifications detected on ultrasound as a marker of malignancy. Laryngoscope 2004;114(10): 1753–7.

15. Danese D, Sciacchitano S, Farsetti A, et al. Diagnostic accuracy of conventional versus sonography-guided fine-needle aspiration biopsy of thyroid nodules. Thyroid 1998;8(1):15–21.

16. Cesur M, Corapcioglu D, Bulut S, et al. Comparison of palpation-guided fine-needle aspiration biopsy to ultrasound-guided fine-needle aspiration biopsy in the evaluation of thyroid nodules. Thyroid 2006;16(6):555–61.

17. Tessler FN, Middleton WD, Grant EG, et al. ACR thyroid imaging, reporting and data system (TI-RADS): white paper of the ACR TI-RADS Committee. J Am Coll Radiol 2017;14(5):587–95.

18. Lauria Pantano A, Maddaloni E, Briganti SI, et al. Differences between ATA, AACE/ACE/AME and ACR TI-RADS ultrasound classifications performance in identifying cytological high-risk thyroid nodules. Eur J Endocrinol 2018;178(6): 595–603.

19. Park SY, Kim E-K, Kim MJ, et al. Ultrasonographic characteristics of subacute granulomatous thyroiditis. Korean J Radiol 2006;7(4):229.

20. Tessler FN, Middleton WD, Grant EG. Thyroid imaging reporting and data system (TI-RADS): a user's guide. Radiology 2018;287(1):29–36.

21. Charous SJ. An overview of office-based ultrasonography: new versions of an old technology. Otolaryngol Head Neck Surg 2004;131(6):1001–3.

22. Slough CM, Randolph GW. Workup of well-differentiated thyroid carcinoma. Cancer Control 2006;13(2):99–105.

23. Podnos YD, Smith D, Wagman LD, et al. The implication of lymph node metastasis on survival in patients with well-differentiated thyroid cancer. Am Surg 2005;71(9):731–4.

24. Zaydfudim V, Feurer ID, Griffin MR, et al. The impact of lymph node involvement on survival in patients with papillary and follicular thyroid carcinoma. Surgery 2008;144(6):1070–7 [discussion: 1077–8].

25. Cunnane M, Kyriazidis N, Kamani D, et al. A novel thyroid cancer nodal map classification system to facilitate nodal localization and surgical management: the A to D map. Laryngoscope 2017;127(10):2429–36.

26. Chan JM, Shin LK, Jeffrey RB. Ultrasonography of abnormal neck lymph nodes. Ultrasound Q 2007;23(1):47–54.

27. van den Brekel MW, Stel HV, Castelijns JA, et al. Lymph node staging in patients with clinically negative neck examinations by ultrasound and ultrasound-guided aspiration cytology. Am J Surg 1991;162(4):362–6.

28. Lesnik D, Cunnane ME, Zurakowski D, et al. Papillary thyroid carcinoma nodal surgery directed by a preoperative radiographic map utilizing CT scan and ultrasound in all primary and reoperative patients. Head Neck 2014;36(2):191–202.

29. Johnson NA, Tublin ME, Ogilvie JB. Parathyroid imaging: technique and role in the preoperative evaluation of primary hyperparathyroidism. AJR Am J Roentgenol 2007;188(6):1706–15.

30. Abboud B, Sleilaty G, Rabaa L, et al. Ultrasonography: highly accuracy technique for preoperative localization of parathyroid adenoma. Laryngoscope 2008;118(9):1574–8.

31. Gurney TA, Orloff LA. Otolaryngologist-head and neck surgeon-performed ultrasonography for parathyroid adenoma localization. Laryngoscope 2008;118(2):243–6.

32. Gofrit ON, Lebensart PD, Pikarsky A, et al. High-resolution ultrasonography: highly sensitive, specific technique for preoperative localization of parathyroid adenoma in the absence of multinodular thyroid disease. World J Surg 1997;21(3):287–91.

33. Ruda JM, Hollenbeak CS, Stack BC. A systematic review of the diagnosis and treatment of primary hyperparathyroidism from 1995 to 2003. Otolaryngol Head Neck Surg 2005;132(3):359–72.

34. Yeh MW, Barraclough BM, Sidhu SB, et al. Two hundred consecutive parathyroid ultrasound studies by a single clinician: the impact of experience. Endocr Pract 2006;12(3):257–63.

35. Steward DL, Danielson GP, Afman CE, et al. Parathyroid adenoma localization: surgeon-performed ultrasound versus sestamibi. Laryngoscope 2006;116(8):1380–4.

36. Lundgren E, Rastad J, Ridefelt P, et al. Long-term effects of parathyroid operation on serum calcium and parathyroid hormone values in sporadic primary hyperparathyroidism. Surgery 1992;112(6):1123–9.

37. Udelsman R. Six hundred fifty-six consecutive explorations for primary hyperparathyroidism. Ann Surg 2002;235(5):665–70 [discussion: 670–2].

38. Stephen AE, Milas M, Garner CN, et al. Use of surgeon-performed office ultrasound and parathyroid fine needle aspiration for complex parathyroid localization. Surgery 2005;138(6):1143–50 [discussion: 1150–1].

39. Abdelghani R, Noureldine S, Abbas A, et al. The diagnostic value of parathyroid hormone washout after fine-needle aspiration of suspicious cervical lesions in patients with hyperparathyroidism. Laryngoscope 2013;123(5):1310–3.

40. Li W, Zhu Q, Lai X, et al. Value of preoperative ultrasound-guided fine-needle aspiration for localization in Tc-99m MIBI-negative primary hyperparathyroidism patients. Medicine (Baltimore) 2017;96(49):e9051.

41. Traxler M, Schurawitzki H, Ulm C, et al. Sonography of nonneoplastic disorders of the salivary glands. Int J Oral Maxillofac Surg 1992;21(6):360–3.

42. Bialek EJ, Jakubowski W, Zajkowski P, et al. US of the major salivary glands: anatomy and spatial relationships, pathologic conditions, and pitfalls. Radiographics 2006;26(3):745–63.

43. Martinoli C, Pretolesi F, Del Bono V, et al. Benign lymphoepithelial parotid lesions in HIV-positive patients: spectrum of findings at gray-scale and Doppler sonography. AJR Am J Roentgenol 1995;165(4):975–9.

44. Isa AY, Hilmi OJ. An evidence based approach to the management of salivary masses. Clin Otolaryngol 2009;34(5):470–3.

45. Haidar YM, Moshtaghi O, Mahmoodi A, et al. The utility of in-office ultrasound in the diagnosis of parotid lesions. Otolaryngol Head Neck Surg 2017;156(3):511–7.

46. Deandrea M, Mormile A, Veglio M, et al. Fine-needle aspiration biopsy of the thyroid: comparison between thyroid palpation and ultrasonography. Endocr Pract 2002;8(4):282–6.

47. Izquierdo R, Arekat MR, Knudson PE, et al. Comparison of palpation-guided versus ultrasound-guided fine-needle aspiration biopsies of thyroid nodules in an outpatient endocrinology practice. Endocr Pract 2006;12(6):609–14.

48. Bohacek L, Milas M, Mitchell J, et al. Diagnostic accuracy of surgeon-performed ultrasound-guided fine-needle aspiration of thyroid nodules. Ann Surg Oncol 2012;19(1):45–51.

49. Graciano AJ, Fischer CA, Chone CT, et al. Efficacy of ultrasound-guided fine-needle aspiration performed by surgeons newly trained in thyroid ultrasound. Head Neck 2017;39(3):439–42.

50. Bellevicine C, Vigliar E, Malapelle U, et al. Cytopathologists can reliably perform ultrasound-guided thyroid fine needle aspiration: a 1-year audit on 3715 consecutive cases. Cytopathology 2016;27(2):115–21.

51. Wu M, Choi Y, Zhang Z, et al. Ultrasound guided FNA of thyroid performed by cytopathologists enhances Bethesda diagnostic value. Diagn Cytopathol 2016; 44(10):787–91.

52. Cappelli C, Pirola I, Agosti B, et al. Complications after fine-needle aspiration cytology: a retrospective study of 7449 consecutive thyroid nodules. Br J Oral Maxillofac Surg 2017;55(3):266–9.

53. Denham SLW, Ismail A, Bolus DN, et al. Effect of anticoagulation medication on the thyroid fine-needle aspiration pathologic diagnostic sufficiency rate. J Ultrasound Med 2016;35(1):43–8.

54. Khadra H, Kholmatov R, Monlezun D, et al. Do anticoagulation medications increase the risk of haematoma in ultrasound-guided fine needle aspiration of thyroid lesions? Cytopathology 2018;19(8):1167.

55. Su P-H, Wang T-G, Wang Y-C. Ultrasound-guided injection of botulinum toxin in a patient with omohyoid muscle syndrome: a case report. J Clin Ultrasound 2013; 41(6):373–6.

56. Kim J-H. Ultrasound-guided sclerotherapy for benign non-thyroid cystic mass in the neck. Ultrasonography 2014;33(2):83–90.

57. Rehrer M, Mantuani D, Nagdev A. Identification of peritonsillar abscess by transcutaneous cervical ultrasound. Am J Emerg Med 2013;31(1):267.e1-3.

58. Nogan S, Jandali D, Cipolla M, et al. The use of ultrasound imaging in evaluation of peritonsillar infections. Laryngoscope 2015;125(11):2604–7.

59. Fordham MT, Rock AN, Bandarkar A, et al. Transcervical ultrasonography in the diagnosis of pediatric peritonsillar abscess. Laryngoscope 2015;125(12): 2799–804.

60. Huang Z, Vintzileos W, Gordish-Dressman H, et al. Pediatric peritonsillar abscess: outcomes and cost savings from using transcervical ultrasound. Laryngoscope 2017;127(8):1924–9.

61. Biron VL, Kurien G, Dziegielewski P, et al. Surgical vs ultrasound-guided drainage of deep neck space abscesses: a randomized controlled trial: surgical vs ultrasound drainage. J Otolaryngol Head Neck Surg 2013;42(1):18.

In-Office Evaluation and Management of Dysphagia

Abdulmalik S. Alsaied, MD*, Gregory N. Postma, MD

KEYWORDS

- Dysphagia • Office-based procedure • Transnasal esophagoscopy
- Flexible endoscopic evaluation of swallowing • High-resolution manometry

KEY POINTS

- Dysphagia is a relatively common complaint; it is considered an alarming symptom that needs further evaluation and a diagnosis.
- The self-administered 10-item eating assessment tool is used to assess the initial patient symptom severity and to monitor the efficacy of management.
- Pharyngeal squeeze maneuver evaluates the pharyngeal muscular strength; it is an important factor in the examination of swallowing.
- Flexible endoscopic evaluation of swallowing is helpful in the identification of penetration, aspiration, residue, and the effectiveness of swallowing compensatory strategies.
- High-resolution manometry is a useful adjunctive study to measure the pharyngeal strength, function of upper esophageal sphincter, lower esophageal sphincter, and esophageal motility.

OVERVIEW

Dysphagia means the sensation of impaired swallowing that can occur at any point from the oropharynx to the gastroesophageal junction, so it is a symptom rather than a diagnosis. Dysphagia can range from an isolated sensation of food being stuck in the throat to a significant swallowing impairment that leads to the dependence on a feeding tube. Dysphagia is considered an alarming symptom, which requires further evaluation.[1] Approximately 20% of the population experiences some degree of dysphagia,[2] with the prevalence further increasing to 50% in individuals older than 65 years.[3] Untreated dysphagia can lead to aspiration pneumonia, lung abscess, or even death. Risk factors for dysphagia include advancing age, history of head and neck cancer, radiation therapy, stroke, neuromuscular disease, or aerodigestive tract

Disclosure Statement: The authors have nothing to disclose.
Department of Otolaryngology, Voice, Airway and Swallowing Center, Medical College of Georgia at Augusta University, 1120 15th Street, Augusta, GA 30912, USA
* Corresponding author.
E-mail address: a.s.alsaied@gmail.com

Otolaryngol Clin N Am 52 (2019) 577–587
https://doi.org/10.1016/j.otc.2019.02.007
0030-6665/19/© 2019 Elsevier Inc. All rights reserved.

tumors. In general, dysphagia to solids suggests an underlying anatomic disorder, whereas dysphagia to liquids often relates to a neurologic disorder.[4]

Dysphagia can be divided into 2 main types: oropharyngeal and esophageal dysphagia. In oropharyngeal dysphagia, patients usually complain of difficulties with initiation of swallowing, passing bolus down to the esophagus, or coughing and choking immediately after swallowing. Cricopharyngeus (CP) hypertonicity and weakness of pharyngeal muscles are classic examples of this type. Esophageal dysphagia symptoms start several seconds after the initiation of a swallow. Esophageal dysphagia could be due to an anatomic defect, such as tumors, strictures, or motility disorders.[1] Often the patient can localize the site of dysphagia, either suprasternal or retrosternal. Typically, suprasternal dysphagia is usually unreliable and could mean oropharyngeal or esophageal disorder. However, retrosternal dysphagia almost always indicates an esophageal pathologic condition.[5]

EATING ASSESSMENT TOOL-10

The eating assessment tool-10 (EAT-10) is a 10-item tool that is self-administered (**Table 1**).[6] It is a validated tool to assess both the initial patient symptom severity and the efficacy of treatment. An EAT-10 score of 3 or more is considered abnormal.

EXAMINATION

During examination, the physician should note the quality of voice. A wet voice can indicate laryngeal penetration, whereas dysarthria suggests a central neurologic disease. Laryngeal elevation may be evaluated during a dry swallow, and gag reflex should be assessed with tongue depressor as well. The patient is asked to cough to assess the effectiveness of this protective mechanism. Flexible laryngoscopy should be performed for evaluation of vocal fold mobility and glottic closure as well as the presence or absence of pooling at the pyriform sinuses or vallecular space.

Pharyngeal Squeeze Maneuver

The pharyngeal squeeze maneuver (PSM) is a clinical evaluation of pharyngeal muscular strength and serves as an important predictor of safety of swallowing.[7]

Table 1 Eating assessment tool-10					
0 = No Problem; 4 = Severe Problem					
1. My swallowing problem has caused me to lose weight.	0	1	2	3	4
2. My swallowing problem interferes with my ability to go out for meals.	0	1	2	3	4
3. Swallowing liquids takes extra effort.	0	1	2	3	4
4. Swallowing solids takes extra effort.	0	1	2	3	4
5. Swallowing pills takes extra effort.	0	1	2	3	4
6. Swallowing is painful.	0	1	2	3	4
7. The pleasure of eating is affected by my swallowing.	0	1	2	3	4
8. When I swallow, food sticks in my throat.	0	1	2	3	4
9. I cough when I eat.	0	1	2	3	4
10. Swallowing is stressful.	0	1	2	3	4
				Total EAT-10:	

From Belafsky PC, Mouadeb DA, Rees CJ, et al. Validity and reliability of the eating assessment tool (EAT-10). Ann Otol Rhinol Laryngol 2008;117(12):922; with permission.

During flexible laryngoscopy, the patient is asked to produce a forceful, high-pitched, crescendo/eee/, while observing for the lateral hypopharyngeal walls contraction and obliteration of the pyriform sinuses. PSM is classified as intact or diminished only. Those with an absent PSM are at significant risk to aspirate.[8]

FLEXIBLE ENDOSCOPIC EVALUATION OF SWALLOWING

Flexible endoscopic evaluation of swallowing (FEES) was first described by Langmore and colleagues[9] in 1988. FEES provides a dynamic evaluation of swallowing with different food consistencies and liquids. It is helpful in detection of penetration, aspiration, residue, and the effectiveness of protective coughs.[7] If abnormal swallowing is observed, FEES has the advantage of the ability to evaluate the effectiveness of bolus consistency modifications and swallowing compensatory strategies, "for example, head rotation posture, breath-holding, or multiple swallows," and assist in making recommendations.[10]

The equipment needed to perform FEES is a flexible endoscope, viewing/recording monitor, different consistencies of testing food materials (water or ice chips, puree, and crackers), and food coloring to help with the identification of the bolus.

Technique

Using nasal local anesthesia during FEES is controversial. Although usage of topical anesthetic nasal spray is part of some protocols, others have concern about alteration of pharyngeal or laryngeal sensation.[7]

The study starts with the patient in a seated position, and the endoscope is passed through the more patent side of the nasal cavity. Soft palate movement and velum closure are evaluated by asking the patient to say /kakaka/. Then, the scope is advanced to have a panoramic view of the hypopharynx and larynx. Swallowing challenge usually starts with water or ice chips; if patient passes, then, pureed consistencies are used. If patient passes the puree, then crackers can be tested. With each tested material, patient is instructed to keep the bolus in his/her mouth and not to swallow immediately. This additional maneuver is to rule out premature spillage, which is the loss of bolus into the hypopharynx before the initiation of swallow.

Occasionally, the order of tested consistency may change. For example, in patients with impaired laryngopharyngeal sensation, swallow challenge starts with puree.[5] In cases of bolus penetration or aspiration during FEES, the penetration aspiration scale (PAS) can be used to quantify the findings (**Table 2**).[11]

Limitations of FEES include the inability of the test to assess the oral phase, base of tongue activity, and hyolaryngeal elevation.

Sensory Testing

Sensory testing is an adjunctive tool to FEES to assess the integrity of laryngopharyngeal sensation. The test is conducted by a brief tactile stimulus to supraglottic mucosa (eg, over the aryepiglottic fold) on one side and observation of the bilateral rapid and brief adduction of vocal folds "laryngeal adductor reflex (LAR)."[12,13] The mucosal stimulus can be delivered either by a light touch with the tip of the endoscope or by calibrated puffs of air through the side channel of the flexible endoscope. The degree of laryngopharyngeal sensory deficit is correlated to the amount of calibrated air puffs required to elicit the LAR. The higher air pressure needed, the more impairment of laryngopharyngeal sensation. A normal individual shows LAR at air pressure of 3 mm Hg. Reflex at 6 mm Hg is considered mild impairment; reflex at 9 mm Hg is considered moderately impaired, and sensations are considered severely impaired if there is no

Table 2 Penetration aspiration scale	
Score	**Description**
1	Material does not enter the airway
2	Material enters the airway, remains above the vocal folds, and is ejected from the airway
3	Material enters the airway, remains above the vocal folds, and is not ejected from the airway
4	Material enters the airway, contacts the vocal folds, and is ejected from the airway
5	Material enters the airway, contacts the vocal folds, and is not ejected from the airway
6	Material enters the airway, passes below the vocal folds, and is ejected into the larynx or out of the airway
7	Material enters the airway, passes below the vocal folds, and is not ejected from the trachea despite effort
8	Material enters the airway, passes below the vocal folds, and no effort is made to eject

From Rosenbek JC, Robbins JA, Roecker EB, et al. A penetration-aspiration scale. Dysphagia 1996;11(2):94; with permission.

reflex triggered at a pressure of 9 mm Hg.[7] Both sides of the supraglottis should be tested. The presence of bilateral sensory impairment is a powerful clinical indicator of poor swallowing.[7]

TRANSNASAL ESOPHAGOSCOPY

Shaker,[14] in 1994, was the first to describe the unsedated transnasal esophagogastro-duodenoscopy with a small-diameter flexible endoscope. This procedure then gained popularity among otolaryngologists following a publication by Herrmann and Recio[15] in 1997 and a live demonstration by Aviv[16] at a national meeting in 1998.

The diameter of transnasal esophagoscopes ranges between 3.1 and 5.3 mm (depending on the model), and a transnasal esophagoscope provides a working channel for suction, irrigation, and air insufflation.

Technique

Adequate topical anesthesia is important to mitigate the patient's anxiety for the procedure. The more patent nasal cavity is sprayed with an atomized 1:1 mixture of topical oxymetazoline and either 2% tetracaine or 4% topical xylocaine for both decongestion and anesthesia. If additional topical nasal anesthetic is needed, this mixture can be applied to cotton pledgets, which are then placed in the nasal cavity for 5 to 10 minutes. Topical anesthetic agent may be sprayed to the oropharynx if desired, or the patient will be asked to gargle and swallow viscous lidocaine, which should be adequate for a diagnostic transnasal esophagoscopy (TNE) and for any esophageal intervention performed. Although adequate anesthesia is essential, excessive anesthesia should be avoided. Should the hypopharynx become overly anesthetized, secretions can be aspirated, which will induce coughing during the procedure. Recent oral intake is not an absolute contraindication for the procedure; however, the patient is advised to take nothing per mouth at least 3 hours before the procedure to decrease the risk of regurgitation and aspiration.[17]

The procedure is done while the patient is in a sitting position; the endoscope is then introduced into the nasal cavity. Once the pharynx and larynx are visualized, the patient is asked to tilt the head down to flex the neck. The endoscope is then held in position just above the postcricoid region. The patient is then asked to swallow to allow for introduction of the endoscope into the esophagus. Air insufflation and suction are used as needed to advance the scope smoothly beyond the lower esophageal sphincter (LES) to the stomach. Air is then insufflated into the stomach, and retroflexion is performed to allow a view of the endoscope passing through the gastroesophageal junction and cardia of the stomach; this is performed by rotating the entire endoscope 180° and maximally turning the endoscope tip 210°. Once a retroflexed view is obtained, the additional air is suctioned from the stomach to relieve the discomfort. The endoscope is then slowly withdrawn, and the distal esophagus is evaluated with attention given to the gastroesophageal junction. The remainder of the esophagus is examined with use of insufflation, suction, and irrigation. The postcricoid region is particularly difficult to fully evaluate and is best visualized by insufflation with a burst of air as the endoscope is withdrawn from the esophagus.

The squamocolumnar junction (SCJ) "Z-line" is located at the meeting of the grayish-white–colored squamous esophageal mucosa with the salmon-colored columnar gastric mucosa. The SCJ normally coincides with the proximal extent of the gastric rugae. If the SCJ is extending above the proximal extent of the gastric rugae, then the diagnosis of Barrett esophagitis is suspected. If Barrett esophagitis or other mucosal lesions or masses are noted during TNE, flexible biopsy forceps are passed through the working channel, and multiple biopsies are obtained. Sliding hiatal hernia can be suspected by the proximal extension of the gastric rugae greater than 2 cm from the diaphragmatic compression. The retroflexed view can help in identification of hiatal hernias. Any benign-looking mucosal lesion should be identified during TNE and monitored (**Fig. 1**).

If difficulty is encountered passing the endoscope through the upper esophageal sphincter (UES), the examiner should suspect the possibility of CP muscle dysfunction or a hypopharyngeal diverticulum.[17]

In cases of suspected foreign body (FB) ingestion, TNE can be implemented as a diagnostic tool to rule out esophageal FB in cases of inconclusive lateral neck radiograph.[18] The flexible forceps can be used through the working channel for esophageal FB removal if needed.[19,20] However, in cases of suspected airway risk, conventional esophagoscopy under general anesthesia and intubation is the procedure of choice.

Guided Observation of Swallowing in the Esophagus

Belafsky and Rees[21] in 2009 described the guided observation of swallowing in the esophagus (GOOSE) examination. GOOSE is performed during TNE by asking the patient to swallow boluses of liquid, puree, crackers, and pills while the endoscope is held in certain positions "above the aortic compression, above the LES, and retroflexed in the stomach." GOOSE can aid in identification of any organic pathologic condition, abnormal esophageal motility, and bolus transit time, taking into account that normal esophageal transit time is less than 13 to 15 seconds.

TREATMENT
In-Office Esophageal Balloon Dilation

In-office esophageal balloon dilation over guidewire with local anesthesia was first described in 2007.[22] Benefits of balloon dilation in-office include low complication

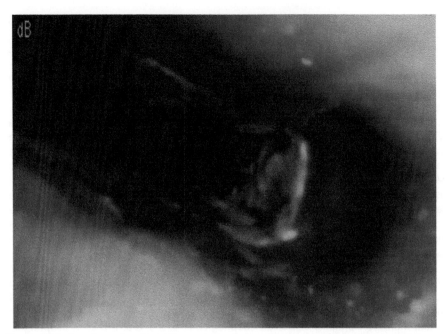

Fig. 1. Pill-induced esophagitis with esophageal ulcer. The patient had a history of tetracycline intake and presented with odynophagia.

rate, avoidance of general anesthesia, and having patient feedback during the procedure. The limitations include patient discomfort and pain, and this procedure requires patient cooperation.[23] Candidates for esophageal dilation are patients with esophageal stricture, ring, or web, and patients with CP muscle dysfunction. It is particularly useful for neopharyngeal stricture after laryngectomy.

Technique
The local anesthesia is similar to that described for TNE. The procedure starts with diagnostic TNE and confirming the pathologic condition; the esophagoscope is kept in the esophagus, and a guidewire is passed through the working channel until it passed beyond the area of interest. The esophagoscope is drawn out while advancing the guidewire until the scope is completely out of patient's nasal cavity. The assistant should hold and secure the guidewire in position while pulling the guidewire all the way through the esophagoscope. The scope is reintroduced from the same nasal cavity until there is a good view of the site intended to be dilated. The proper size balloon is advanced over the guidewire and into the patient. The midpoint of the balloon should be positioned exactly over the area intended to be dilated to guarantee the maximum effect. Inflation of the balloon and dilation are started progressively until resistance is encountered and then held for 30 to 60 seconds. Then, the balloon is deflated while advancing (this is to keep the esophageal segment open for better visualization and evaluation for mucosal tears).

"Superdilation" (dilation with 2 balloons side by side) can be done by the same technique, except that passing the guidewire will be done 2 times (both in the same nostril) (**Fig. 2**).

Upper Esophageal Sphincter and Lower Esophageal Sphincter Botulinum Toxin Injection

There are 7 different serotypes of botulinum toxin identified; however, only 2 of them are available for clinical use, type A and type B. Type A has a longer duration of effect and less diffusion from the injection point compared with type B. In the authors' institute, botulinum toxin type A (Botox, Allergan, Irvine, CA, USA) is used, which is considered in this article. Botulinum toxin specifically binds to the acetylcholine-releasing presynaptic nerve terminals, subsequently inhibiting the release of acetylcholine into neuromuscular junctions, which leads to reversible chemical denervation and temporary muscle paralysis.

Upper Esophageal Sphincter Injection

The UES is a 2- to 4-cm high-pressure zone separating the distal pharynx from the proximal esophagus. The most important component of the UES is the CP muscle, which is a C-shaped muscle attached to the lateral aspects of the cricoid cartilage without a median raphe. It makes up the lower 1 to 2 cm of the UES.[24] The CP muscle receives innervation from the pharyngeal plexus and the recurrent laryngeal nerve as well.[4]

The CP muscle is active and contracted at rest and relaxed during swallowing. Impaired or uncoordinated relaxation of CP muscle is called CP dysfunction, which can be caused by several conditions, for example, stroke, Parkinson disease, amyotrophic lateral sclerosis, increased acid reflux, and postradiation therapy for head and neck cancer, or it may be idiopathic.[25]

Schneider and colleagues[26] were the first to describe Botox injection into the CP muscle as a nonsurgical treatment option for CP dysfunction. Patients with impaired CP muscle relaxation but having intact pharyngeal muscle strength and hyolaryngeal elevation are good candidates for CP muscle botulinum toxin injection.[4] The dose used ranges from 15 to 100 units and depends on patient age, dysphagia severity, and the presence of feeding tube. In young patients with severe CP dysfunction and

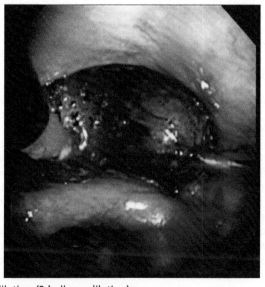

Fig. 2. UES superdilation (2-balloon dilation).

a preexisting feeding tube, the dose can be as high as 100 units; older patients with mild CP dysfunction may receive an initial dose of 15 units. Then, future dosing can be adjusted according to the response. The effect starts within weeks of injection and lasts up to 5 to 6 months on average. Botox should be prepared in small volume and high concentration to minimize the risk of diffusion of toxin into the other surrounding muscles.[23,25] Diffusion of botulinum toxin can cause worsening dysphagia if the toxin diffuses into the pharyngeal muscles, or less commonly but serious, respiratory distress if posterior cricoarytenoid muscles are affected. In cases of severe adverse effects of Botox injection, Pyridostigmine (peripheral acetylcholinesterase inhibitor) can be used as an antidote, to safely reverse the effect of botulinum toxin.[27]

Technique

In-office CP muscle botulinum toxin injection can be done either transcervically with electromyography (EMG) guidance or via the flexible endoscope with the flexible needle (flexible 23-gauge × 200-cm sclerotherapy needle, Injection Therapy Needle Catheter; Boston Scientific, Marlborough, MA, USA). The transcervical approach with EMG guidance depends on the unique CP muscle signal, which is electrically active at rest, relaxes with swallowing, and does not change with sniffing or phonation.

The flexible endoscopy with the flexible needle technique starts with TNE and identification of the CP muscle. The flexible needle is primed with the botulinum toxin dilution and passed through the working channel. Then, the intended dose is injected at 3 points in the CP: 1 posterior and 2 laterally.

Lower Esophageal Sphincter Injection

Rees[28] described botulinum toxin injection into the LES with the aid of TNE. Indications for this procedure include achalasia, distal esophageal spasm, and nutcracker esophagus.

Technique

This procedure starts by performing a diagnostic TNE; then, the LES (gastroesophageal junction) is localized in the standard method. An amount of 100 units of botulinum toxin is diluted in 4 mL of injectable saline. The entire volume is drawn into a 5-mL syringe, so 1 mL of air is added to the syringe to compensate for the dead space in the long injection needle. Under direct visualization, the toxin is injected at 8 sites (0.5 mL per site) in the LES.[27]

HIGH-RESOLUTION MANOMETRY WITH IMPEDANCE

High-resolution manometry (HRM) is a useful tool to measure pharyngeal strength, and the function of UES, LES, and esophageal motility. Impedance describes the transport function of the esophagus using a liquid bolus.

The solid-state HRM with impedance catheter typically has 36 circumferential sensors spaced 1 cm apart, and 18 intraluminal impedance sensors spaced at 2-cm intervals. The catheter's diameter is 4.2 mm. The data obtained are presented by using pressure topography color plots (**Fig. 3**). The current indications for esophageal HRM include diagnosing primary and secondary esophageal motility disorders; further evaluation of symptoms, such as "dysphagia, noncardiac chest pain, or globus sensation"; evaluation of refractory acid reflux; diagnosing the anatomic abnormalities like hiatal hernia; evaluation of esophageal function before therapeutic surgical interventions; assessment of esophageal obstruction in post-fundoplication patients; and when combined with impedance, evaluation for the association between esophageal motility disorders and esophageal transit.[29]

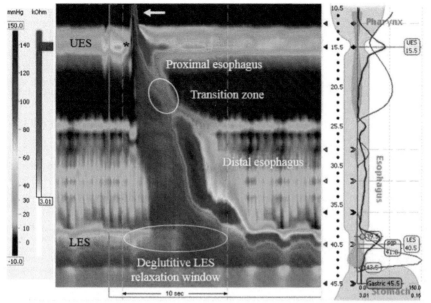

Fig. 3. Pressure topography color plots of normal swallow in a normal subject. Time is on the horizontal axis, and the length of the catheter is on the vertical axis (centimeters from nares). On the left is the pressure scale encoded in colors; the red color end reflects the high-pressure zones, and the blue end indicates the low-pressure regions. The purple color plot in the study indicates the transport (impedance) along the catheter sensors. Note the complete relaxation of the UES (*asterisk*) and normal hypopharyngeal pressure wave (*arrow*). The transition zone demarcates the minimal pressure zone, which is located between the striated muscle of the proximal esophagus and the smooth muscle of the distal esophagus. The onset of the deglutitive relaxation window is defined by the onset of upper sphincter relaxation, and it lasts either 10 seconds or until the arrival of the peristaltic contraction. UES is located 15.5 cm from the nares, and the LES is located at 40.5 cm. (*Courtesy of* Combined high-resolution esophageal impedance-manometry. ManoScan ESO Z; Medtronic, Shoreview, MN).

The test is done in a sitting position. The study protocol is that after the insertion of the catheter transnasally there is a 5-minute assessment of UES and LES baseline function followed by the evaluation of 10 swallows (5 mL of water each swallow).

In CP dysfunction, the classic HRM findings are elevated UES residual pressure and elevated hypopharyngeal intrabolus pressure as well. The characteristic HRM findings in achalasia are incomplete LES relaxation and absence of esophageal peristalsis. Scleroderma typically shows preservation of the proximal esophageal peristalsis with weak or absent distal peristalsis, associated with a hypotensive LES. When there is ≥50% ineffective swallows detected in the HRM, ineffective esophageal motility is considered.[30]

SUMMARY

There are many different evaluative and diagnostic studies that can be done in the office-based setting to assess patients with dysphagia. In selected cases, these procedures are effective, safe, and cost saving.

REFERENCES

1. Ferguson DD, DeVault KR. Dysphagia. Curr Treat Options Gastroenterol 2004; 7(4):251–8.
2. Cho SY, Choung RS, Saito YA, et al. Prevalence and risk factors for dysphagia: a USA community study. Neurogastroenterol Motil 2015;27(2):212–9.
3. Meng NH, Wang TG, Lien IN. Dysphagia in patients with brainstem stroke: incidence and outcome. Am J Phys Med Rehabil 2000;79(2):170–5.
4. Kuhn MA, Belafsky PC. Management of cricopharyngeus muscle dysfunction. Otolaryngol Clin North Am 2013;46(6):1087–99.
5. Kuhn MA, Belafsky PC. Functional assessment of swallowing. In: Johnson J, editor. Bailey's head and neck surgery: otolaryngology. Volume. 57. Philadelphia: Lippincott Williams & Wilkins; 2013. p. 825–37.
6. Belafsky PC, Mouadeb DA, Rees CJ, et al. Validity and reliability of the eating assessment tool (EAT-10). Ann Otol Rhinol Laryngol 2008;117(12):919–24.
7. Merati AL. In-office evaluation of swallowing: FEES, pharyngeal squeeze maneuver, and FEESST. Otolaryngol Clin North Am 2013;46(1):31–9.
8. Bastian RW. Videoendoscopic evaluation of patients with dysphagia: an adjunct to the modified barium swallow. Otolaryngol Head Neck Surg 1991;104(3): 339–50.
9. Langmore SE, Schatz K, Olsen N. Fiberoptic endoscopic evaluation of swallowing safety: a new procedure. Dysphagia 1988;2:216–9.
10. Leder SB, Murray JT. Fiberoptic endoscopic evaluation of swallowing. Phys Med Rehabil Clin N Am 2008;19(4):787–801.
11. Rosenbek JC, Robbins JA, Roecker EB, et al. A penetration-aspiration scale. Dysphagia 1996;11(2):93–8.
12. Aviv JE, Martin JH, Keen MS, et al. Air pulse quantification of supraglottic and pharyngeal sensation: a new technique. Ann Otol Rhinol Laryngol 1993; 102(10):777–80.
13. Aviv JE, Martin JH, Kim T, et al. Laryngopharyngeal sensory discrimination testing and the laryngeal adductor reflex. Ann Otol Rhinol Laryngol 1999;108(8):725–30.
14. Shaker R. Unsedated trans-nasal pharyngoesophagogastroduodenoscopy (T-EGD): technique. Gastrointest Endosc 1994;40(3):346–8.
15. Herrmann IF, Recio SA. Functional pharyngoesophagoscopy: a new technique for diagnostics and analyzing deglutition. Oper Tech Otolayngol Head Neck Surg 1997;8(3):163–7.
16. Aviv JE. Transnasal esophagoscopy: state of the art. Otolaryngol Head Neck Surg 2006;135(4):616–9.
17. Johnson CM, Postma NG. Transnasal esophagoscopy. In: Flint PW, Haughey BH, Robbins KT, et al, editors. Cummings otolaryngology-head and neck surgery. Amsterdam: Elsevier Health Sciences; 2014. p. 1020–4.
18. Shih CW, Hao CY, Wang YJ, et al. A new trend in the management of esophageal foreign body: transnasal esophagoscopy. Otolaryngol Head Neck Surg 2015; 153(2):189–92.
19. Abou-Nader L, Wilson JA, Paleri V. Transnasal oesophagoscopy: diagnostic and management outcomes in a prospective cohort of 257 consecutive cases and practice implications. Clin Otolaryngol 2014;39(2):108–13.
20. Bennett AM, Sharma A, Price T, et al. The management of foreign bodies in the pharynx and oesophagus using transnasal flexible laryngo-oesophagoscopy (TNFLO). Ann R Coll Surg Engl 2008;90(1):13–6.

21. Belafsky PC, Rees CJ. Functional oesophagoscopy: endoscopic evaluation of the oesophageal phase of deglutition. J Laryngol Otol 2009;123(9):1031–4.
22. Rees CJ. In-office unsedated transnasal balloon dilation of the esophagus and trachea. Curr Opin Otolaryngol Head Neck Surg 2007;15(6):401–4.
23. Venkatesan NN, Belafsky PC. Office-based treatment of dysphagia. Oper Tech Otolayngol Head Neck Surg 2016;27(2):104–13.
24. Sivarao DV, Goyal RK. Functional anatomy and physiology of the upper esophageal sphincter. Am J Med 2000;108(4):27–37.
25. Sulica L, Blitzer A. Botulinum toxin treatment of upper esophageal sphincter hyperfunction. Oper Tech Otolayngol Head Neck Surg 2004;15(2):107–9.
26. Schneider I, Thumfart WF, Pototschnig C, et al. Treatment of dysfunction of the cricopharyngeal muscle with botulinum A toxin: introduction of a new, noninvasive method. Ann Otol Rhinol Laryngol 1994;103:31–5.
27. Young DL, Halstead LA. Pyridostigmine for reversal of severe sequelae from botulinum toxin injection. J Voice 2014;28(6):830–4.
28. Rees CJ. In-office transnasal esophagoscope-guided botulinum toxin injection of the lower esophageal sphincter. Curr Opin Otolaryngol Head Neck Surg 2007; 15(6):409–11.
29. Pandolfino JE, Kahrilas PJ. AGA technical review on the clinical use of esophageal manometry. Gastroenterology 2005;128(1):209–24.
30. Kahrilas PJ, Bredenoord AJ, Fox M, et al, International High Resolution Manometry Working Group. The Chicago classification of esophageal motility disorders, v3. 0. Neurogastroenterol Motil 2015;27(2):160–74.

Moving?

Make sure your subscription moves with you!

To notify us of your new address, find your **Clinics Account Number** (located on your mailing label above your name), and contact customer service at:

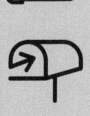

Email: journalscustomerservice-usa@elsevier.com

800-654-2452 (subscribers in the U.S. & Canada)
314-447-8871 (subscribers outside of the U.S. & Canada)

Fax number: 314-447-8029

Elsevier Health Sciences Division
Subscription Customer Service
3251 Riverport Lane
Maryland Heights, MO 63043

*To ensure uninterrupted delivery of your subscription, please notify us at least 4 weeks in advance of move.